Child Sexual Abuse
Informing practice from research

David PH Jones
*Consultant Child and Family Psychiatrist and Honorary Senior
Lecturer, Park Hospital for Children, Oxford*

and

Paul Ramchandani
*Specialist Registrar in Child and Adolescent Psychiatry,
Park Hospital for Children, Oxford*

Foreword by
Lady Elizabeth Butler-Sloss

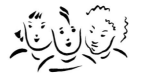

Radcliffe Medical Press

Radcliffe Medical Press Ltd
18 Marcham Road, Abingdon, Oxon OX14 1AA

British Library Cataloguing in Publication Data

A catalogue record for this book is available from the British Library.

ISBN 1 85775 362 3

Typeset by Acorn Bookwork, Salisbury, Wilts.
Printed and bound by Hobbs the Printers, Totton, Hants

Contents

Foreword by Lady Elizabeth Butler-Sloss

Over the last ten to fifteen years both the professionals and the public have become increasingly aware of the existence of child sexual abuse and of its serious effect upon its young victims. Much has been written on the cause of sexual abuse and on the most effective protective and preventative measures to put into place in the multi-disciplinary approach to the issues raised by it. One problem is the communication gap between the valuable research already available and the day-to-day practice of the front-line practitioners faced with enormously difficult problems and often without the resources or the time to seek out and absorb that research. The Department of Health have been in the forefront of seeking the best practice and communicating it to practitioners countrywide. With a grant from the Department, the authors of this book have drawn on research findings to answer questions about each stage of the protection process to which they have added their own invaluable commentary. I noted with particular interest the investigation into associated problems for a child who has been sexually abused, the importance of comprehensive assessment and planning which stresses the involvement and participation of the family and the implications of the research findings for the practitioners.

Each chapter of this book sets out at the beginning questions and issues and at the end a most useful summary entitled 'Implications for practitioners'. Although designed mainly for social workers and mental health practitioners, in my view it ought to have a much wider reading public, including judges, barristers and solicitors engaged in family law.

Elizabeth Butler-Sloss
Royal Courts of Justice, London
January 1999

Acknowledgements

This project was funded by a grant from the Department of Health, and undertaken at the University of Oxford Section of Child and Adolescent Psychiatry.

It was undertaken with the help of an advisory group, to whom we express our gratitude. The members of this group were:

Jenny Gray
Chair
Social Services Inspectorate, Department of Health

Jane Aldgate
Professor, School of Social Work, University of Leicester

Christine Ballinger
Area Manager – Children and Families, Social Services Department, Dudley

Arnon Bentovim
Consultant Child Psychiatrist, London Child and Family Consultation Service

Carolyn Davies
Senior Principal Research Liaison Officer, Department of Health

Elaine Farmer
Research Fellow, School for Policy Studies, University of Bristol

Ann Gross
Section Head, Social Care Group 3A, Department of Health

Andy Hampson
Principal Officer Child Protection, Salford Social Services Department

Jill Hodges
Consultant Child Psychotherapist, Great Ormond Street Hospital, London

Robert Jezzard
Senior Policy Adviser, Department of Health

Helen Jones
Social Services Inspector, Department of Health

Elizabeth Monck
Independent Consultant, London

Ian Rush
Director of Social Services, Trafford Metropolitan Borough Council, Manchester
Association of Directors of Social Services

David Skuse
Professor of Behavioural Sciences, Institute of Child Health, University of London

Marjorie Smith
Deputy Director, Thomas Coram Research Unit, London

Judith Trowell
Consultant Child and Adolescent Psychiatrist, Tavistock Clinic, London

We also thank others who provided helpful comments, particularly Willma Bartlett, NSPCC child protection training officer; John Geddes and members of the Department of Psychiatry, University of Oxford; Lucy Berliner, Sexual Assault Centre, Seattle; Gill Nineham of Radcliffe Medical Press.

Finally and most importantly we thank Jenny Gray, Social Services Inspector at the Department of Health, who commissioned the work, and encouraged and advised us throughout.

Although this book is the result of ideas generated by a large number of people, the final responsibility for this work rests with the authors.

Chapter 1

Introduction

In this book we identify and summarise selected key research findings on intervening with sexually abused children, their family members and alternative carers. These have implications for practitioners, their managers, and planners and commissioners of services. Throughout, we have emphasised an evidence based approach to this crucial work. Research should support practice, not dictate it, and the hope is that this review will aid practitioners in their work. The best use of research is to examine it critically for oneself and take out the messages that are most helpful to practice. We hope that this review will facilitate this process for practitioners and their managers.

When a child is identified as having been sexually abused it is rarely found to be the sole problem, and a range of co-existing family based difficulties is a common finding. Problems such as domestic violence, parental mental illness, substance abuse, and parenting problems including physical abuse and neglect, pose additional challenges for effective intervention. However, not all child victims are abused within families, many being abused by known but trusted figures within the neighbourhood or in out-of-home care. In these circumstances too, coexisting difficulties abound. The cost of not intervening is great in terms of damaged development, personal difficulties for the abused child in adult life and, for some, the move to being an abuser of other vulnerable children.

There is no simple theory or model with which to explain either the occurrence or the consequences of child sexual abuse. However, there are frameworks that can prove helpful. The 'developmental ecological' perspective, widely accepted, is particularly useful. It is explained in detail elsewhere, but briefly it has two broad themes, developmental and ecological, as follows.[1-3]

The first is the developmental one, which stresses that the child becomes increasingly organised, integrated, yet more complex as an individual as he or she grows up.[4] There are many influences on this process, amongst them genetic, physical, psychological, and family influences, as well as wider neighbourhood and cultural influences. Traumatic events, such as child sexual abuse, can lead to disruption and derailment of the process of normal development. Subsequent influences on the child can either be ameliorating or further potentiate the effect of early damage.

The second theme in this model is the ecological one. This considers the child within their environment surrounded by layers of successively larger and more complex social groupings, which have an influence on him or her. These include the family and extended family, friendship networks, school, neighbourhood, and work influences, and the family's place within the community. Still wider is the influence of the culture within which the family live. These are shown in Figure 1. As well as this, both the child and their parent influence the outcome of events via their personalities and social functioning.[5] In fact, parents have one of the greatest relative influences within this model.

Several important implications flow from this perspective. One is that dissimilar pathways can arrive at similar destinations in terms of the effect upon the developing child, and conversely similar pathways can have quite diverse outcomes. Secondly, the perspective reflects the understanding that development is a process which involves interactions between the growing child and his or her social environment. Thirdly, while the experience of a phenomenon such as child sexual abuse can damage a child's development, change is still possible in many different ways. Therefore, the range of positive and negative influences are important to consider

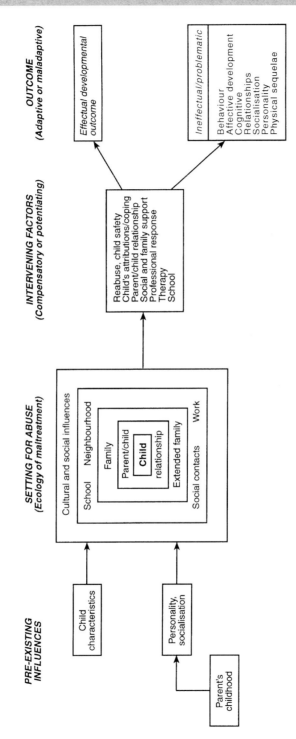
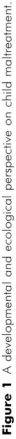

Figure 1 A developmental and ecological perspective on child maltreatment.

when examining the occurrence, or looking at the outcome, of an influence upon children, such as sexual abuse.

Once abuse has occurred, there are a number of intervening factors which influence outcome. These include the individual child's coping skills and strategies, parental and family support, and societal influences including the impact of child protection procedures and, where offered, psychological treatments. Each of these factors may have a beneficial effect or may worsen outcome for the child and their family. It is these intervening factors, and particularly the child protection process and psychological treatments, that we focus on in this book, with the aim of helping practitioners and their managers achieve the best outcome for sexually abused children and their families.

Methodology

Our aim has been to gather together the currently available research (both published and unpublished) and to draw out those key findings which have relevance to those professionals working with children and families where a child has been sexually abused.

In deciding how far to search for evidence we divided the area up into two (*see* Figure 2). The first covers broad issues in child protection, including the formal child protection process, and the contextual setting within which this operates. The second area focuses particularly on psychological treatments. We have adopted a differing approach to the way in which we have searched for and included studies in the two areas.

1 The child protection process

The system of child protection practice varies from country to country around the world. Whilst some similarities exist, the differences can be large. As a consequence, we have focused on literature from the United Kingdom when considering this area, as this seemed of most relevance to UK practitioners. In this we have drawn largely on the research initiated

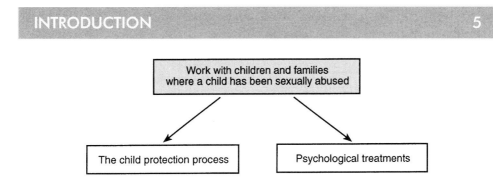

Figure 2 Methodology: dividing the process.

and funded by the Department of Health as part of the 'Studies in Child Protection' series.[6-17] Good quality research into the UK system of child protection has been sparse, and the included studies constitute a large proportion of this. Not all of these studies focus exclusively on sexual abuse, but where possible we have drawn out those findings that pertain particularly to this form of abuse.

2 Psychological treatments

In recent years there have been notable trials conducted examining therapeutic help for children and families following disclosure of child sexual abuse. These have predominantly been conducted in the United States, although there have been some UK based trials. In searching for trials in this area we have attempted to include all the treatment studies which are of a randomised controlled or controlled design. As a starting point we have used the excellent review of Finkelhor and Berliner.[18]

From there we have searched Medline and other bibliographic databases using standard searching methods in collaboration with librarians in Oxford.[19] We have retrieved references from papers and books and contacted principal researchers and experts, both in the United Kingdom and the United States. We have examined abstract books from recent international conferences. From these efforts we have gathered and read a wide range of material.

Appraising the evidence

We have critically appraised each individual study for its methodological strengths and limitations in order to be able to place appropriate weight and confidence on its findings. To do this we have used standard critical appraisal formats, the exact one depending on the study design. For quantitative studies we have used the 'Users' Guides' developed at McMaster University,[20] and for qualitative studies we have used the guidelines prepared for the *Journal of Evidence-Based Mental Health*.[21,22] This has given us a firm basis for extracting key relevant findings for this publication.

Strengths and limitations of this book

As we have critically appraised the research, it seems only fair that we should be explicit about the strengths and weaknesses of our own work in this book.

This is not a summary based on all the available evidence. Given a time limit, choices have had to be made about the most fruitful sources of information. In our writing about treatment options we feel we have overcome this as far as is possible by searching thoroughly for all available controlled trials. However, there are other areas of practice which we have not been able to address fully, either because the research evidence is lacking, or because of limitations of space. One area we have excluded is the important field of work with abusing adults and juveniles, as this fell outside the remit of our study. Another important omission is a consequence of the way in which issues such as ethnicity, culture and learning disability are not addressed thoroughly by the bulk of the research. This means that within this review we are unable to discuss these issues as fully as they warrant given their key importance within the context of child protection.

Any research, particularly in the qualitative field, must consider issues of bias. We are both medical practitioners, and inevitably this will influence the topic areas of particular interest to us. We have tried to overcome this by using standardised selection and appraisal criteria for the projects we have studied, and by checking our criteria and appraisals with the authors of the original research studies. In addition, we have looked particularly for findings that are consistent across studies.

The review does cover a mixture of qualitative and quantitative research. We have tried throughout to give a clear indication of the weight which we can put on the findings. This has not always been possible, given that this is a small book designed to be easy to read. We have included in the summaries of the research projects what we feel are the main strengths and limitations of each project, and we hope you will read these as an important part of the book (Appendix B). The studies are all referenced at the end and, for those with sufficient time, are the best source to search for information relevant to your own practice.

Despite these caveats we believe that this review represents an important step forward in improving the accessibility of research findings and so making practice as effective as possible. We hope that it will be helpful to front-line practitioners, and consequently of benefit to the children and families they work with.

Any comments you have to make on our work would be welcome. Please write to either of us at: The Park Hospital for Children, Old Road, Headington, Oxford OX3 7LQ.

Organisation of the messages

Each chapter is structured in a similar way:

1 The first box gives a brief summary of the main Questions and issues in this area.

2 The following text describes the key relevant findings from the research we have appraised (The findings).

3 The Comment section represents our own views on the research findings, their implications for practice, and links with other research.

4 The Practice implications box at the end of each chapter
summarises the essential implications for practitioners.

We have endeavoured to separate the research findings from
our own, and others', opinion – whether based on clinical
experience or other research findings, so that the reader can
decide for himself how much weight to place on each chapter.

The pattern of this book broadly follows the child protection
process outlined in *Working Together under the Children Act,
1989,*[23] as illustrated in Figure 3.

One aspect of the child protection process which does not
appear to be addressed by the research we have studied is the
area of immediate protection and planning the investigation.
This lack has been discussed by others and is perhaps a reflec-

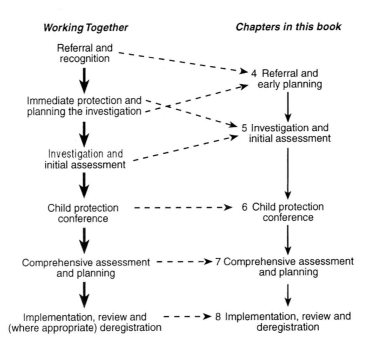

Figure 3 *Working Together under the Children Act, 1989* and the corresponding
chapters in this book.

tion of the difficulty of studying social workers and their decision making as they go about their day-to-day work.[24] As a consequence, we have amended the chapters of this book to correspond more closely to the child protection process as it is described in the research. The corresponding chapters can be easily seen in Figure 3. Despite this, the findings from the research frequently do not easily fall into defined categories, as the process is a fluid one. We have endeavoured to allocate the important research findings to the appropriate chapter, but some overlap and repetition is inevitable.

We have found that, in addition to the areas of the child protection process outlined above (and in Figure 3), the research had much to say about issues such as background factors in cases of child sexual abuse, and treatment issues. We have included these findings, and the chapters that follow fall under the following headings:

- Background (family) factors in child sexual abuse
- Associated problems for a child who has been sexually abused
- Referral and early planning
- Investigation and initial assessment
- Child protection conference
- Comprehensive assessment and planning
- Implementation, review and deregistration
- Psychological treatments
- Measuring outcome.

Chapter 2

Background (family) factors in child sexual abuse

Questions and issues

- To what extent is the finding that a child has been sexually abused embedded within other background or associated problems which also might have an impact on the child's welfare? If so, is this a frequent occurrence?

- Are the families of sexually abused children distinguishable from other families?

- What do we know about those children and their families where the abuser was not a household member?

- Do the parents and siblings of sexually abused children have specific needs and problems that need to be addressed?

- Do cycles of abuse, passing from generation to generation, occur? If so, can anything be done to prevent this occurring?

The findings

Child sexual abuse is frequently associated with other problems, which also affect children's welfare. These are important, not just because of their deleterious effects on child health, but also because of their importance to case planning, treatment and intervention. Although most of the research projects were not specifically designed to look at background factors, several of them do have information about this. Nearly half the families in one study[8] had multiple problems (chronic ill-health, unemployment, poor housing and other forms of abuse occurring), with the high rates of comorbid physical and emotional abuse confirmed in another study.[13] Domestic violence either was or had been a feature in about half the families studied.[9,17] Witnessing or experiencing this intra-familial violence may be a particular risk factor that predicts boys who may go on to sexually abuse others.[15,16] Not all of the child sexual abuse cases looked at by the research were intra-familial. Although there were differences between the studies on what constituted intra- and extra-familial abuse, the associated factors described in this section were occurring in both groups.

Up to one-third of parents, particularly mothers, had experienced problems in their own childhood – particularly sexual or physical abuse,[17] and half of the mothers reported depression when completing screening questionnaires.[13]

The families of children who had been abused were found to be functioning in a more dysfunctional way than comparison families, where the child had not been abused.[17] Using a standardised family assessment measure, the particular problem areas were: less open or direct styles of communication, problems managing their children's behaviour, and less emotional closeness or warmth expressed than in equivalent families where children had not been sexually abused.

Comment

The fact that child sexual abuse (CSA) is closely linked to other potentially noxious influences should not surprise us, but is amply illustrated by the Department of Health Research Studies. A narrowly focused child protection response to CSA, in isolation, is therefore likely to miss other problems that will be necessary to address. Research on the impact of CSA has emphasised the importance of the context within which CSA occurs, as well as the subsequent events during the remainder of childhood, and the links to eventual mental health outcome in adult life.[25]

The aim of intervening in CSA must be to stop abuse recurring, and to render the child safe, but also to provide help for the child's distress and to prevent long-term harm and cycles of abuse recurring in the future. Otherwise, such children are likely to be denied the opportunity for reasonable adjustment in adolescence and adult life, in terms of mental health and the capacity for satisfying relationships with others, including their own children. For all of these reasons the background and accompanying contextual factors surrounding CSA deserve greater attention than they have received thus far, particularly as the focus of service shifts from child protection only to addressing the child's needs more comprehensively.

The findings concerning differences in family functioning are of interest, and have been noted by another group of researchers too,[26] as well as clinicians.[27,28] These authors found that rigid family belief systems, dysfunctional adult partnerships, parental neglect and unavailability, and inability to nurture autonomy in their children characterised sexually abusing families compared with equivalent, but non-abusing families. This is of major significance for mental health services, regardless of whether the observed dysfunction preceded or developed after the sexual abuse. It is particularly important because the dysfunction applies to extra-familial sexual abuse, as well as intra-familial. Up to now, extra-familial cases have typically not received services,[29] as the focus of concern has been the abuse, not the other accompanying problems, including family functioning. Once again these findings underline the importance of the shift from focusing on the abuse alone to a broader appreciation of the child's context and needs.

It is clear that many parents, particularly mothers of sexually abused children, have needs of their own, with many of them having experienced abuse of various types. Successfully addressing these needs is one of the essential tasks of the child protection intervention, not only for the parent, but indirectly for the child, whose needs for care the parents are likely to have to meet.

Practice implications

Assessments of sexually abused children need to be broadly based in order to pick up the range of likely child and family problems which will need to be addressed.

The wider, contextual problems (e.g. domestic violence, other types of maltreatment) can be incorporated into the case planning for cases registered as 'at risk of', or 'actual sexual abuse'.

Addressing family problems and dysfunctional ways of communicating probably helps to prevent poor outcomes in terms of the child's future welfare, as well as recurrence of cycles of abuse.

Families of children abused outside the household often have substantial unmet needs, and even when safe from the extra-familial abuser, are unsafe from other problems that affect their welfare. These problems may be amenable to intervention at the time when the crisis of child sexual abuse brings the child and family into contact with professional agencies.

Chapter 3

Associated problems for a child who has been sexually abused

Questions and issues

- Child sexual abuse (CSA) is an event, or series of events, which happen to a child, rather than being a mental health problem *per se*. However, to what extent is CSA a phenomenon associated with a number of mental health difficulties for the child and his/her family?

- Are there specific patterns of emotional and behavioural problems that occur following sexual abuse?

- How common is sexualised behaviour in children who have been sexually abused?

- Are there characteristic ways in which children and young people cope with being sexually abused? If so, do these coping styles assist or can they cause problems too?

The findings

Mental health

About half of the children studied, who had been sexually abused, experienced depression, post-traumatic stress disorder (PTSD) or disturbed behaviour or a combination of these.[13,14] Those who are removed from home during an investigation may have even higher rates of these problems.[9] Of those young people studied in substitute care 59% admitted to having suicidal thoughts, and two-thirds had high scores for emotional and behavioural problems.[10]

These findings have been confirmed in a controlled study.[17] Sexually abused girls had much higher rates of many psychiatric diagnoses, particularly PTSD, depression and generalised anxiety, than non-abused girls. They also frequently had multiple problems occurring together, including those listed above together with social phobia and reactive attachment disorder.

The same study also looked at ways of coping used by the girls and found that the sexually abused girls were more likely to use distraction, blaming others, resignation and particularly social withdrawal as coping behaviours.

Sexualised behaviour

Sexually abused young people may subsequently show sexualised behaviour,[13] putting them at risk in the future. In a study of 40 sexually abused or abusive children placed in substitute care (both foster care and institutions), four of the girls studied became pregnant and seven children were thought to be involved in prostitution.[10] Sexualised behaviour is also associated with worse health for the young person, in the form of depressive symptoms and somatic complaints.

Sexually abusive behaviours (also called 'interpersonal sexual behaviour problems') were also displayed by some of these children.[10] Many of those children who subsequently abused others had been previously abused themselves (50% in one study).[13] Despite this, and the other sexualised behaviours mentioned above, little therapeutic work is usually done to tackle these concerning and threatening behaviours.[10]

Comment

It comes as no surprise that children who have been sexually abused have high rates of associated psychological problems.

The importance of this finding, however, is that unless an assessment of a child's needs addresses issues such as depression, anxiety, post-traumatic stress symptoms, coping mechanisms and sexualised behaviour, then any comprehensive plan will fail to address them – leaving the child with significant unmet needs. This wide range of, often coexisting, potential problems presents a significant challenge for the assessment of needs and comprehensive planning for effective interventions. It also means that there are significant prevention opportunities at this early stage.

The problem of sexualised behaviour is of deep concern,[30,31] leading as it does to increased potential risk, both for the sexually abused child and, in some cases, risk for other young people, as abused children can develop sexually abusive behaviour/interpersonal sexual behaviour problems. It can be a difficult issue to deal with, both for parents and professionals, and as the research suggests, it is often an issue left unaddressed.[10] However, there are assessment tools available to quantify sexualised behaviour[32] (see Chapter 10), and, increasingly, there is evidence that sexualised behaviour may be channelled and 'treated', at least in younger children.[33]

The problem of interpersonal sexual behaviour problems, as well as personally directed sexual behaviour problems, becomes more important for adolescents, especially those in substitute care.[30] Farmer and Pollock[10] have stressed the potential which exists for preventive work with young people in substitute care concerning sexualised behaviour, interpersonal sexual relationships, and personal safety. This is particularly poignant because of their bleak outcome findings for the sexually abused young people in the care system.

The developmental perspective, described in Chapter 1, emphasises the adaptation of children to their life experiences, including sexual abuse. There is increasing interest in the coping mechanisms and the attributions which sexually abused children develop in the wake of their experiences. We do not yet know whether the coping styles which appear effective at one time remain effective strategies for children as they grow older. Similarly, we cannot yet say how individual children might evolve and change their coping strategies over time, if indeed they do. It is also known that social and environmental influences, such as the availability of support from friends and family members, seem to have an effect on the individual child's coping strategy. Some research has emphasised that active and social coping styles are effective for children.[34,35] Equally, however, the same work found that children who used avoidant coping strategies appeared to obtain short term benefit from them, despite the commonly held view of practitioners who advise against such strategies. Nonetheless, interrelationships between the child's method of coping and the social support which is available to them have received support from several studies.[34,35] Thus, children who receive better support from a parent, and this can be either mothers or fathers, appeared more likely to develop positive attributions concerning their own abuse. One important method of coping is to seek out social support from positive, non-abusive adults. Another important method of coping, associated with positive benefit in both studies of children who have been sexually abused as well as adult survivors, is that of cognitive processing of the traumatic events. Those individuals who were able to think about and make sense of their experiences had relatively better outcomes.[34,36] This links with findings from other researchers who have studied the individuals' perspective and style of appreciation of any traumatic experiences which have happened to them during childhood. They have found that those adults who were, on the one hand, dismissive of the salience of childhood maltreatment or, at the other extreme, overly preoccupied and absorbed with their childhood experiences are the ones who do less well in adult life, compared with those who are able to achieve a more balanced appreciation of their childhood experiences.[37]

These findings have major implications for treatment services. In the first place, unitary, isolated sexual abuse treatment services are unlikely to be able to meet the variety of needs of this population of children and young people.

Rather, a range of services and professionals will be required if this variety of consequences is to be managed effectively. All these services would need to be committed to the issues of safety and child protection and be able to operate within legal frameworks, while respecting the need for multi-disciplinary and multi-agency work. At the individual level, children's coping strategies appear to be positively affected by the social support from positive parental and adult influences which they are able to access. It would appear that the child's coping mechanism must be respected, including avoidant styles which may not be as negative as some practitioners believe. Assisting the child in developing a view of his/her own abuse which avoids the extremes of either overt dismissal of or, on the other hand, an obsessive preoccupation with their abusive experience seems an appropriate objective.

Practice implications

Assessments should incorporate enquiry about mental health problems.

Screening tools may be useful, especially those focusing on commonly found groups of symptoms, so that cases requiring further services can be identified at an early stage.

Management plans for child sexual abuse should incorporate mental health needs which have been identified.

Early identification and treatment of interpersonal sexual behaviour problems/sexually abusive behaviour is an important part of assessment.

The child's coping strategies should be identified, and ways of addressing problematic ones incorporated into the treatment plans.

Chapter 4

Referral and early planning

Questions and issues

- Who refers, and what happens when they do?

- Do referrers obtain the help and responses that they hope for?

- Does early planning occur; and does it involve a range of professionals in strategy discussions – including specialist advisers where needed (e.g. learning disabilities, sensory impairments, and mental health problems)?

- Which professionals take the primary role in responding to referrals?

- Can we recognise the serious sexual abuse cases which need immediate protection because they are in danger, having disclosed secret information?

The findings

The importance of the early contact with the child protection system has been highlighted in many of the studies. In one study,[11] over half of the small sample of children who were placed on the register had been referred by their own mothers. In cases like this, where mothers made the referral, their expectations were often that their children would receive some form of help. This expectation seems to have been greatly disappointed in most cases as protection issues over-shadowed all other needs which the child or other family members had.[9]

Those cases where the referral was made without a carer's knowledge had risks attached too. Parents were not informed about their child being interviewed in up to 75% of those cases under joint social services and police investigation.[9] This secrecy may have jeopardised trust and consequently later care.

Many of the children referred, even for concern about sexual abuse, did not end up being seen by professionals – seemingly on the basis of an evaluation (without face-to-face contact) about the current safety of the child, rather than on whether abuse occurred or not.[14] Some of these children were suspected of, or were at risk of, being abused.

Early planning in cases was often rushed by pressure of work, and professionals seemed not to expect any extra time for more thorough planning of an investigation. We found no evidence in the research about the involvement of specialist advisers at this stage, whether for children with learning disabilities, sensory impairments, or other specific issues.

Little information was available from the studies about the initial investigative interview in cases of suspected sexual abuse. Although it seems that joint investigative interviews have been the norm for some time, in one of the studies [14] nearly one third of these interviews were conducted by the police, without a social worker involved.

Comment

The source and detail of each referral will be different and will of course greatly influence the planning and response, ranging from an immediate response resulting in removal of a child to safety, to a more considered period of information gathering and inter-agency liaison. There can be no uniform response to this problem. It is well to remember, however, that these differing circumstances will also include the expectations of parents. As Farmer and Owen[9] have shown, many parents anticipate receiving help, not the investigation and suspicion which is often perceived to be the normal response of agencies.

Although a limited amount of research has been conducted we do not have a great deal of information on precisely what the professional does on receipt of a referral:[38] what phone calls or checks are made or whether there are strategic planning meetings as to how to approach the prospective investigation. We also have very little information on who leads the investigation – the police or social workers? Without this baseline information little can be said on such crucial issues as how social workers and others make the decisions that they do, and what they base their decisions upon.

Parton[24] has commented on this dearth of information in his critique of *Child Protection: messages from research*.[39] Many of the projects were either ethically or practically constrained, as suggested by this initial, crucial work. However, it is probable that there has been an increase in the number of interviews led by police officers relative to social workers since this research was conducted,[38] due to the subsequent introduction of the *Memorandum of Good Practice* in October 1992.[40]

The recognition of sexual abuse and the various definitions of what sexual abuse is and what is normal sexual behaviour fall outside the remit of this review, but are discussed further in *Child Protection: messages from research* (pp 11–22),[39] which summarises the research of Smith et al.

It seems likely that social workers and police officers will be involved in deciding whether a referral constitutes the likelihood of sexual abuse or not. It does seem that many referrals are dismissed from the child protection system, even at this early stage, often because there is insufficient information upon which to initiate an investigation, or because the decision is made that the complaint is insufficiently substantive to even constitute potential sexual abuse.[14,41] We do not have detailed information as to why front-line practitioners decide not to proceed with up to a quarter of the referrals which are received,[41] nor do we know how many of these rejected referrals come back into the system at any later stage in subsequent years. However, the experience of practitioners suggests, and indications from studies corroborate, that some of these rejected referrals do subsequently appear as substantive cases. Whether they could have been detected and successfully identified at an earlier stage is currently unknown.

The indications from the studies are that cases of suspected sexual abuse are being routed through the child protection system, and being investigated and subsequently conferenced appropriately, once they are within the system.[41] The research does not indicate that cases which are described as 'in need' are being inappropriately described as sexual abuse cases, in order to obtain services. This problem appears to be more of a concern for cases of neglect and less serious physical abuse. However, as we shall see subsequently, children who have been sexually abused do have unmet needs which emerge later on in the child protection process.

The *Memorandum of Good Practice*, although principally focused on the needs of the Criminal Justice System, does contain clear guidance about the planning necessary before an interview with the child is conducted.[40] There is a dearth of information, either from studies within the Criminal Justice System or from the studies which we have reviewed, as to how these planning processes and decisions are actually made in day-to-day practice, although from other sources it seems that planning has been very variable, ranging from no plans through to the making of very detailed plans, prior to interviewing the child.[38]

The lack of involvement of other specialists or persons with specific expertise to assist with the evaluation of child maltreatment and unmet needs of particular groups of children and families is of great concern. For example, specialists from the field of disability, including learning disabilities and sensory communication problems, child mental health specialists, and those with special knowledge of particular minority ethnic or cultural groups or refugees deserve mention, because the research studies on the child protection system have relatively little to add about their contribution. We do not have studies which evaluate the benefit of their addition so much as ones that highlight their absence.

Practice implications

It is important to attempt to work in partnership with parents, especially with mothers (usually the non-abusive caretaker) who refer many, if not most, cases of suspected sexual abuse.

Parents, and especially mothers, require clear information in an attempt to work as openly as possible, in order to keep them engaged with the process.

Informing parents as swiftly and as completely as possible after children have been interviewed is necessary to enable trust to be maintained. Parallel sessions interviewing children and parents in tandem may prove useful.

If conflict occurs between potentially jeopardising the partnership with parents and on the other hand fully protecting the child from harm, it is clear that the child's needs are paramount.

Few specialists are currently involved and thus it may be useful to identify cases that need specialist help at an early stage, for example, interpreters for children with sensory impairments (hearing and vision), other appropriate specialists for children with severe psychiatric problems or learning disabilities.

The early planning stage, following the initial referral, would be the most useful point to identify issues of race, culture or language which may require addressing.

Chapter 5

Investigation and initial assessment

Questions and issues

- How do professionals manage the dilemma of discovering whether a child is safe, while also not alienating potential carers, who may eventually work in partnership with the professional?

- Are professionals able to communicate with all children who are referred to them?

- Is it possible to establish working links with parents in cases where child protection assessments are being conducted?

- What approaches to children or parents are the most successful?

The findings

The way in which a case is handled initially can affect the entire subsequent process. Where handled well and sensitively, keeping the non-abusing parent informed and involved, there can be a positive effect on the eventual outcome. Conversely, poorly handled initial contact can alienate both the child and carer, making later work more difficult.[14] Unsurprisingly, this has been associated with a worse outcome for children. This variation in initial approach may reflect an individual worker's underlying beliefs about the way in which the investigation should be carried out. In a survey of professionals there were two different viewpoints.[6] One group started interventions with parents on the basis of supportive acceptance. The other preferred an approach which required parents to accept responsibility. Most social workers in this particular survey favoured the latter approach.

The initial interview is often difficult, and this can be compounded when there are additional communication problems, for example where a child has learning disabilities or there is not easy access to interpreting services for children whose first language is not English. The development of a computer assisted interview[7] holds promise, particularly as different modules are available in languages other than English (including sign language). The modules also aim to facilitate communication between a child and an interviewer where a child has particular needs such as learning disabilities or attention problems.

The wide range of parental reactions to sexual abuse allegations were often difficult to interpret accurately, particularly where these had to be evaluated at the time of considering placement issues.[14] There was a wide difference in perspectives between the professionals and the parents.[8] Parents were typically shocked, frightened, or became withdrawn, whereas for the professional this was a 'routine' job. In these circumstances professionals sometimes misjudged parental capacity to understand allegations or protect their children. This gap was often at its widest at the time of the initial contact, particularly in cases where sexual abuse was suspected but not clear-cut. Parents were often afraid that their child would be taken away, even when this was not on the professional's agenda.[14]

Comment

The crucial importance of the initial contact has been emphasised by many of the Department of Health projects.

The fact that the quality of the early or initial contact affects later working relationships with professionals should not really surprise us. However, what might is that, despite the child protection focus of the initial professional response, both children and their parents held expectations of help being received. Hence, they remained receptive and wanted assistance despite initial difficulties. This was an encouraging finding, lending hope that even if the initial contact presents difficulties for practitioners, the prospect of working in partnership is not lost for ever, because the children and mothers appear to remain open to help with their predicament. This is important because, although the call for partnership has obvious and immediate appeal to all humane practitioners, it is sometimes extremely difficult to sustain during the initial crisis occasioned by the revelation of sexual abuse.

The issue of initial contact in the field of CSA is complicated by its nature. In particular, secrecy, deception and admonitions 'not to tell' are hallmarks of CSA cases; hence, open methods of working with full expectations of honest responses from parents can be ill-advised. When you do not yet know what you are going to face, how can the initial contact with the child and family be done in such a way as to give the child the best opportunity to talk, if he or she wishes to, while at the same time avoiding alienating parents who may well provide future support and care? Supportive contact with the non-abusive parent (whose very identity may not be apparent to begin with) will be crucial to outcome.

The dissonance between the viewpoints of the professionals and the parent caught in the immediate aftermath of the revelation of sexual abuse is a finding with clear implications for professionals. The potential for misinterpretation in these circumstances is great, as are the implications for effective supervision of front-line practice. The practitioner faces the difficult task of balancing the need to obtain the non-abusing parent's commitment to help protect the child, while also being responsive to that parent's needs for understanding, information and psychological treatment.[42] The evidence points to the benefits of focused, psychoeducational approaches to this task, by a sympathetic worker who seeks a partnership with the parent in distress.[14,43] Is it possible for a supportive and accepting stance to co-exist with an approach that encourages parental acceptance of responsibility? Some practitioners hold that these are not dichotomous choices, but instead a tension which can be usefully maintained, while a non-abusive parent negotiates and overcomes the shock of initial discovery.[2]

Other work has confirmed that children are particularly sensitive to professionals who treat them personally, with care, and above all with respect.[42,44,45] Not surprisingly, they want to be informed about the purpose of the process that they are going through, and not be pressured or have their views and attitudes discounted, merely because of the fact that they are children.

These studies record what people think after an event, rather than events as they are occurring. Most case records are not fully contemporaneous, so it is necessary to exercise caution about the extent to which these reflect actual events, or *post-hoc* perceptions and memories. Some studies have attempted to match the views of consumers of services with those of practitioners, revealing points of both dissonance and agreement.[8,14] Nonetheless, as memories they are significant in themselves, for it is upon these that future relationships with direct workers will be founded. The research messages also underline the importance of discussing the perceptions and feelings of parents and children openly, as the course of the investigation unfolds, so that the potential support of the non-abusive caretaker can be harnessed.

Practice implications

The initial approach is extremely important and sets the tone for the remainder of the investigation.

Parents found that professionals who treated them personally, with care and respect, and who listened to their perspectives and were generally non-judgemental were the most help.

Children were especially sensitive to being patronised or kept in the dark, and wanted information and openness from the practitioner.

There is a need for specialist help to be available for minority ethnic children or those with particular needs.

It may be hard to evaluate the potential for a parent to be supportive to his/her child, and easy to misinterpret the parent's first reactions. This may require further evaluation by the professional in order to clarify parental reactions and responses.

In cases where partnership is initially difficult with parents, perhaps because of the need to take immediate child protective action, it may still be possible to work in partnership despite early difficulties.

Parents benefit from direct information and instructions as to how best to help and respond to their child, particularly when they themselves are in a state of crisis and have reduced coping ability as adults.

Chapter 6

Child protection conference

Questions and issues

- In what circumstances are child protection conferences held?

- Are sexual abuse cases relatively more likely to be registered than other types of abuse? If so, why?

- What occurs in conferences? What are the principal activities and outcomes?

- Do we know what factors influence decision making?

- Are parents and children involved?

The findings

Children were more likely to be subject to a child protection conference if the sexual abuse was considered to have been within the family, the case was already an open case prior to referral, and where parents were adjudged unsupportive to their children. The decision to hold a conference was not linked to the professionals' views as to the certainty about whether the abuse had occurred, nor linked to severity of abuse.[14]

Once conferenced, children were more likely to be placed on the Child Protection Register if the abuse occurred within the family rather than outside. Registration appeared to bear little or no association with other case or family characteristics.[14]

Much of the research about child protection conferences from the Department of Health's 'Studies in Child Protection', which were summarised in *Messages from Research*,[39] was conducted around the time of the introduction of the government guidance, *Working Together under the Children Act, 1989* in 1991.[23] At this time, assessment of risk and the decision about whether to register the child(ren) or not took up most of the time at child protection conferences. This left little time to discuss the child protection plan – an average of 9 minutes in one study[9] – so decisions about assessments of needs and case management were given less prominence,[9,14] and often had to be taken by the key worker at a later time.

A number of different factors affected the level of concern expressed when a case of suspected abuse was discussed at a child protection conference. Some of these were related to the professionals involved, and some were case related. Professionals varied widely in the degree of concern they expressed about a particular case of suspected abuse. This was explored in a study using a series of case vignettes.[6] The professions at the two extremes were social workers and health visitors, with health visitors expressing most concern, and social workers the least. This may be a reflection of the day-to-day exposure to cases of abuse which social workers experience. Also, long exposure to a case can raise a professional's threshold of concern, making them less likely to respond to deterioration in the child's situation.[8]

Case-related factors that affected levels of concern included the type of abuse. Cases of physical and sexual abuse were rated as more severe than emotional abuse or neglect.[6] There were also higher levels of concern expressed in a case vignette where the family was black than in the same case where the family's race was not mentioned. Some children and families, particularly those deemed not to have been abused or to have been abused by an outsider, did not receive any further services after the initial investigation.[14]

Two out of three professionals invited to child protection conferences attended. Social workers, police, health visitors, school nurses and principal social workers were the most frequent attenders,[11] with general practitioners being the most frequent non-attenders of those invited. The non-attendance of key professionals was a major concern of the professionals surveyed.[6]

Parents and children felt marginalised if they were not kept informed in the period prior to a conference.[9] Parental attendance was sparse in the studies (parents were at only three of the 48 conferences studied),[11] although there was some variation from region to region.[8] Professionals surveyed generally supported parental attendance, with 66% thinking parents should be able to attend for part of the conference. Only 14% thought that parents should be able to attend all of a conference.

Comment

Some things about the child protection conference have changed since this research was conducted. For example, it is probable that parental attendance has increased considerably, in the wake of the work on increasing parental participation.[43] It is possible that this has led to changes in the proportion of the conference devoted to discussion of the child protection plan, although recent Social Services Inspectorate reports would still question this assumption.[46] It is also possible that there remains a discrepancy between the local policy and the nature of actual practice. Nonetheless, it remains the case that the explicit purpose of the conference is to consider registration, and secondly to construct a child protection plan if need be. It still appears that the focus on planning is very much secondary. This may be a lost opportunity, for a multi-disciplinary group gathered to discuss an individual child and family is a rare event, and an opportunity for making immediate plans to protect the child and initiating core group working.

An assessment of whether significant harm has occurred and/or may occur in the future is a key function of the child protection conference. It is central to decisions about registration and any decisions about the initial child protection plan. The variability between different professionals' level of concern, assessment of potential harm, and the variability dependent on case-related factors, including race, do need further exploration in order to understand fully their origin in decision-making sequences. However, the recent Department of Health materials on assessment[47] and the evaluation of needs, including protection, combined with the training initiatives which are planned to follow their introduction may well help to overcome some of these difficulties. Additionally, it is hoped that these materials will help professionals identify family situations requiring services other than immediate child protection, through the identification of the full range of needs of the individual child and family.

Certain groups, however, were much less likely to be conferenced in the first place, far less registered. One such group are those children sexually abused by other children whilst in substitute care, to whom we will return later (see pages 45–6). A further group that stands out are those sexually abused children abused by persons outside the family. These cases are not only filtered out of the child protection system but out of the Social Services department, with the result that an understanding of their full range of needs is missed and appropriate services do not follow. The reason that such cases are not brought into the child protection conference, and potential registration system, is because the children are not perceived to be at risk of repeat sexual abuse. Whilst the decision not to hold a child protection conference may be appropriate, this presumption about the children's future welfare can be an erroneous one for professionals to make, as there is evidence that children sexually abused outside their family do have significant rates of reabuse. This is presumably because of more subtle vulnerabilities or continuing disturbances in their family environment.[48] However, in addition to the possibility of repeat sexual abuse, children who are abused outside the family have a greater chance of being subject to other forms of abuse, neglect, and parenting difficulties than comparison children.[49-52] Hence, the identification of extra-familial sexual abuse provides an opportunity for identification of the wider needs of this particular child and family. Once again, the fact that children and families' social work practice has become so focused on index instances of child maltreatment and immediate protection results in the wider needs of children becoming subsumed by the priorities and imperatives of child protection.[24]

The non-attendance of important involved professionals is of concern. It may be that reconsidering the timing and siting of conferences will overcome this to a degree, but non-attendance is likely to remain a problem for some professionals. The collection of these professionals' opinions and views on the case under discussion might be aided by use of a standard form. Similarly, the conference needs the input of professionals who can contribute specialist skill and knowledge where this is necessary (e.g. children with sensory impairments, learning disability, or mental health problems). We have already noted that such expertise could be beneficial in the early stages of recognition and planning, but they are important here to assist with the evaluation of needs, including protection needs, and case planning.

We have little information on how the potential dangers of an abusive parent's participation in the child protection process can be dealt with. The issues of children being exposed to reprisal, or mothers exposed to subsequent domestic violence as a consequence of split loyalties, are issues which have probably become more prominent since the increase in participation in conferences by parents, carers, and children themselves.

There are clearly potential difficulties when a group of professionals from different disciplines and perspectives, with varying perceived and actual degrees of persuasion and influence, come together to discuss children and parents. The group processes involved have been noted,[53] but not recently systematically studied, although it is likely that these will affect decision making.

The overriding message from the studies reviewed is that the focus on registration has detracted from case planning for the overall needs of the index child and his/her family. The government's intention to alter this balance in favour of emphasising the child protection plan and desired outcomes for improving the child's welfare is congruent with these findings.[54]

Practice implications

New assessment materials are being designed to overcome some of the variability in practice which currently exists concerning the decision to have a conference, or to register.

Conference and registration depends on obtaining the views of all involved with the child and family. Thus ways of overcoming non-attendance, and involving other specialists appropriately, need to be found.

Multi-disciplinary child protection conferences are key opportunities for establishing core group working and planning interventions. Thus, the time devoted to these activities justifies equality with considerations over registration.

It may be important for participating parents and children to see the focus on intervention and possible outcomes, rather than concentration on registration alone.

Parental participation in conferences considering child sexual abuse needs particularly careful planning, especially where the full extent of the abuse, and degree of involvement of different family members, is not yet known. Additionally, the extent of accompanying domestic violence or other forms of coercion, threat and violence may not be fully appreciated at the point of the initial child protection conference.

Chapter 7

Comprehensive assessment and planning

Questions and issues

- Are comprehensive assessments carried out on children who are on Child Protection Registers?

- Do children and families have access to the child protection plan?

- Do they know what is required of them and what needs to change?

- Which professionals are centrally involved in case planning – do they form 'core groups'?

- What do plans contain: treatment plans? Risk assessments?

The findings

Once a child has been registered, the initial child protection plan is formulated in the conference – the first aspect of which should be the undertaking of a comprehensive assessment.[23] Formal assessments were not the norm for many children who were considered sexually abused, although they were more likely in cases that were subject to conferences and formally registered.[14]

Where registration occurred the most frequently mentioned intervention listed was social worker input. Health resources, such as the health visitor and child and family psychiatry, were less frequently used.[11] Doctors, including paediatricians and psychiatrists, were often seen as difficult to collaborate with by other involved professionals.[11] The use of inter-agency working dropped away as the intervention progressed, usually leaving the social worker with the case. In a few instances 'core groups' of professionals were set up, which could prove helpful.[11] These most commonly included social workers, health visitors, teachers and education welfare officers. Support and good supervision for social workers left holding cases was an integral part of the work in some studies.[12,17] However, many social workers have felt unhappy with the quality of their supervision,[9] particularly given the stressful and wide range of tasks that had to be undertaken.[14]

Parental commitment to the plan could be lacking (although in the studies they had rarely been involved in the drawing up of the child protection plan). This could manifest itself as them not attending follow-up appointments arranged with health staff, or not participating in other aspects of the plan.[11]

Comment

Comprehensive assessment and planning was not a consistent feature of these cases, despite the clear need. The Social Services Inspectorate have noted that where such assessment and planning has occurred, it has been supported by clear procedural requirements and relevant resources.[46] Their analysis of the inspections which they undertook between 1992 and 1996, examining all forms of maltreatment, was that most assessments were incomplete, and practice was inconsistent and often lacking focus. There were insufficient details about the roles and responsibilities of the different professionals and no clear objectives for work. This overall picture was found in the studies of sexual abuse cases reviewed here. Several aspects of this problem were noted. One was the

tendency for the momentum to leave cases after the child
protection conference. Social workers are often left carrying
cases alone, which does not seem appropriate, given the
breadth of unmet needs, and the complexity and attendant
stress of working with sexual abuse cases. However, we note
that mechanisms for encouraging core group working, identi-
fying and harnessing a small group of key front-line professionals with each particular case, have evolved since the
original research was conducted. A linked theme was the
need for effective supervision of casework, not merely with
respect to case management but also on the handling of
complex relationships with clients (children, adults, abusers,
non-abusers), and the direct work being undertaken by front-
line social workers and others. In line with these observations,
the lack of professionals and individuals with specialist
knowledge for a particular case was a theme throughout these
studies. When the broad range and variety of needs presented
by these cases is considered, it is hardly surprising that case
management proves difficult if only one professional is
involved and taking a leading role with the case. Different
perspectives of the various family members will need to be
considered, especially the non-abusive caretaker (most
frequently mothers). Several studies have found that unless
mothers in these circumstances are engaged and feel that
their perspectives are appreciated by the professional
network, they are less likely to follow up with future appointments and arrangements to be engaged in the care plan for the
child. This perspective is taken up later, under treatment (*see*
pages 54–5).

In a number of respects, the difficulties noted with a lack of
comprehensive assessment and planning are linked to the
relative absence of focus on the child protection plan within
the child protection conference itself (*see* page 38). Thus, if
the stage is not set for a focus on planning to meet the needs
of the child and family, but is instead focused on registration
and the index, identified form of maltreatment, then it follows
that the interests of professionals, parents and others who
could assist the child tend to wane. For it is the attendance of

both professionals and parents that has been noted to decline in the period after the initial conference.

Practice implications

Comprehensive assessments, systematically evaluating the available information, are crucial to the success of case planning. Hence, the relevant resources and procedural requirements are necessary for their success.

A multi-disciplinary approach, involving other professionals and agencies as well as social workers in a core group of front-line practitioners, appears to be the best model for meeting the needs of abused children and their families.

Parents need to be involved and participate as fully as possible in the child care plan. This is important, even in those cases where their participation in the process of registration itself is difficult.

Effective supervision and support for front-line practitioners working with abused children and their families is not just desirable, but essential.

Chapter 8

Implementation, review and deregistration

Questions and issues

- Are children kept safe through child protection?

- Are child protection plans implemented and reviewed?

- Are unmet needs of children and families identified and, if possible, plans made to meet their needs?

- Are the mental health needs of children identified where they occur – emotional states, conduct and sexual behaviour problems?

- Are the needs of sexually abused children in substitute care identified and responded to?

- Does case review occur and if so, does it result in desired outcomes for children?

The findings

1 Protection from reabuse

The safety and protection of the child has been at the heart of the protection process in recent years. However, a large number of children remain vulnerable despite professional intervention. In one study of sexually abused children, a half of all children seen were considered vulnerable to further abuse three months after referral. Nearly one in five was considered definitely unsafe at one year after referral.[14] These estimates were based on a researcher's point of view, but they receive support from one of the other research projects which examined all forms of abuse.[8] Sixteen of the 61 children studied were reabused during follow-up.

2 Follow-through plans and unmet needs

Child protection plans were not always implemented, particularly with regard to intervention and therapeutic work.[14] However, the process of holding conferences and registering children did improve their chances of receiving follow-through services,[14] although in another study, review meetings to assess progress had only happened in just over half of the cases.[11] Nonetheless, follow-through services for sexually abused children were more likely to be delivered if the abuse was more certain, more severe in type, and perpetrated by a family member.[14] There is a suggestion from the research that the focus of professional concern may broaden to a more comprehensive response, encompassing the child's and family's needs, as time progresses,[14] but this is not a consistent finding.

There have been five main problems identified in monitoring the implementation of child protection plans: (1) poor recording in social work notes, (2) lack of parental cooperation in some cases, (3) a change in the case or child's circumstances, (4) lack of resources, and (5) lack of ongoing inter-agency work and cooperation.[11]

A consistent finding across the studies has been the large numbers of children who, following sexual abuse, do not get offered, or do not receive therapeutic help. An association between getting therapeutic help and improved behaviour was reported for those children in the care system, who are often the most troubled.[10] But only 20% of the sexually abused children in that study were offered any form of formal psychological help or counselling. In another study of sexually abused children, one-half of those not getting treatment were still depressed three months later.[14] Children who were abused by adults outside the family seemed at particular risk of missing out on any further treatment, as their safety was often assured, so their other needs were over-looked.[14]

Sexual abuse had a high impact on families in the studies.[17] Parents had to cope with their children's distress and with their own distress and guilt feelings. Their own needs at various stages following abuse allegations were often not met. In one study, 75% of parents were in poor psychological health at three months, although this tended to improve over time.[14] Parents had wide-ranging emotional reactions, which were often difficult for workers to interpret correctly.[14] These needs of the parents were often ignored or overlooked, and little support offered to non-abusing parents.[9] In some cases, parents did not even know when their child's case had been closed.[14] Both child and parent(s) had differing and changing needs as time progressed following the abuse. Some needs, particularly psychological needs, were not immediately apparent, and could only be discovered with later repeated assessments.[14]

Overall, there seemed to be a low proportion of cases where there was a successful conviction.[9] This often led to the abused child feeling badly let down when hopes had been raised by professionals and family members. Failure to prosecute an abuser who was a family outsider was associated with a poor outcome for both the child (who was depressed) and his/her parent (who remained unengaged).[14]

3 Substitute care

Sexually abused children were sometimes placed away from home because of the abuse. However, many of those in substitute care who had been sexually abused were placed in care for reasons other than the sexual abuse which they had suffered.[10] In some cases this may have been because the abuse was revealed after they had been placed. Up to a quarter of girls in one study were in some form of substitute care – either foster care or institutional care.[17] Those in care were likely to have suffered longer abuse at the hands of more perpetrators than those who remained at home.[10,17] Unsurprisingly, they were also more depressed.[9]

Despite the vulnerability of many of these children placed in substitute care, the mix of children with whom they were put in a potential placement was often not considered fully. One study found evidence of the types of children in a placement and their histories of abuse or abusing being considered in only nine of their 40 cases.[10]

Substitute care can be a place of further risk to these young people. Some may be exposed to other young people with abusive pasts. Despite this, when cases of abuse did arise in the context of substitute care, they were often not referred to the police for investigation, and the abused and abusers were often not offered therapeutic help.[10]

Comment

Reabuse and persisting vulnerability to abuse at follow-up is clearly a major concern as an outcome for a process purporting to protect children. The detailed reasons for this persisting vulnerability and lack of safety are not fully explored in the studies, but there are several pointers to a link with a lack of follow-through services. We do not know whether, if such services had been available, the children would be less vulnerable to reabuse and persisting difficulties, because the broader context of deprivation, social disadvantage and poverty is likely to have enduring influence despite more services. However, the significant links of persisting and even worsening child depression with continuing lack of safety and vulnerability to reabuse serves to underline the need for support services, direct social work and psychological treatments to be integrated for individual cases. Also, we note that while reabuse and persisting vulnerability may be the case for sexual abuse, it is also present for other forms of maltreatment – physical abuse and neglect – emphasising the value of a comprehensive assessment of background difficulties and coexisting problems, so that a comprehensive picture of a child's needs is obtained.

The unmet needs for information, education, support and specific psychological help are highlighted in several studies, again emphasising the requirement for some basic needs including social support to be met, combined with psychological treatment aimed at both children and family members. These needs are especially likely to remain unmet in cases involving sexual abuse from outside the family. Here, because of the initial focus on abuse and protection, the child's and family's needs for direct social work and other specialised inputs remained unmet, because there appeared to be no adequate machinery to assess, plan and implement services for these families. However, within those cases that *were* brought into the system, through conferencing and registration, there were encouraging signs that the focus of assessment and case planning did broaden from protection only to a broader response to need. Nonetheless, it seems that this did not necessarily meet the perceived needs of children or their parents.[14]

The focus on the most severe and intra-familial varieties of sexual abuse is understandable in terms of the preoccupation of social work services in deciding when to intervene in family life, but the research message does seem clear, namely that the focus of concern, assessment, case planning and delivery needs to broaden from child protection alone to a broader appreciation and response to the child's and family's needs. This applies whether the index cause for concern consists of sexual abuse within or without the family.

Inspections have revealed a variable pattern of practice, with little evidence as to whether core groups have met or plans been implemented, plus a notable lack of time scales against which to audit the progress or otherwise of a family.[46] Statutory case reviews were being held on time, however, and quality improved during the period 1992–96. Deregistration practice was showing a similar improvement. It was noted that the increasingly constrained financial climate was having a negative impact on the available services, particularly health services.[46]

The research does underline the needs of those children with interpersonal sexual behaviour problems. Their needs remain unmet, particularly within substitute care placements. The fact that the needs of children and families change over time underlines the requirement of an ethos of continuing assessment rather than one of single 'risk assessment'. This may be particularly important as the lexicon of risk assessment gains momentum, bringing with it the false hope that through this process risk can be managed. What is required is the resources and spirit of inter-agency working, combined with procedures and the will to follow cases through, keeping assessments alive and adapting services to the needs of children and their families.

The special requirements of substitute care placements for sexually abused children were brought into relief by these studies. In many ways this is a neglected area of study, yet contains the more severely disadvantaged, and severely sexually abused children.[55] The low status of work in the residential care arena, combined with a dearth of foster care placements which are geared up to respond to the particular demands of the children and young people who have been sexually abused, is emphasised here. Care itself can pose additional risks for children who are already vulnerable. There are innovative programmes which are focused on this particular group of sexually abused children, and this seems particularly important when consideration is given to the significant number of vulnerable young people who leave the care system and go on to have serious problems in late adolescence and early adult years. In terms of prevention, and reducing cycles of continuing maltreatment and parenting difficulties, this group deserves special attention.

The findings concerning the low proportion of cases where there was successful conviction of abusers are echoed in the more recent studies of the impact of implementing the *Memorandum of Good Practice*.[40] This implementation occurred in October 1992, after the majority of data for these Department of Health studies were collected. Both the Social Services Inspectorate[38] and the University of Leicester team[56] emphasised the relatively low rate of prosecution in these cases, despite the introduction of videotaped interviews as well as a series of other legislative changes which were designed to allow more evidence from children in criminal cases involving sexual abuse. However, the research in this series of studies is echoed by the findings by two US studies, both of which emphasise the adverse impact on the abused child and the non-abusive caretaker when the prospect of criminal prosecution is initially enthusiastically promised, but not ultimately delivered.[57,58] The UK studies have emphasised the connection between the sense of let down on the one hand, and poor outcome in terms of children's mental health and the engagement and capacity to work in partnership with the non-abusive carer (usually mothers). Perhaps the focus on criminal prosecution has jeopardised child welfare; if so, the balance will require redressing.

Practice implications

Continuing comprehensive assessment linked to service provision is needed rather than one-off assessments of risk, because the needs of sexually abused children and their families change over time.

Children's and families' needs are broad, and so assessment and services cannot be restricted to child sexual abuse alone.

Mechanisms are needed for inter-agency and inter-professional follow-through plans to occur.

Plans need to be specifically linked to outcomes with time scales, so that reviews can focus on progress or its absence.

Both intra-familial and extra-familial cases have substantial needs for assessment and services.

Sexually abused children in substitute care deserve special focus because of the severity of their problems, range of needs, and implications for their future development.

Chapter 9

Psychological treatments

Questions and issues

- Does psychological treatment help to improve the outcome for sexually abused children?

- Which sexually abused children are in need of and would respond to psychological treatments? Should this include all sexually abused children, or merely the symptomatic?

- How specialised or focused should treatment be? Should treatment be orientated towards specific symptoms, or towards child, family, non-abusing parent, abuser, or all of these?

- What do we know about 'sleeper effects', or different types of presentation at different developmental stages? How long should sexually abused children be followed up?

- Which psychological treatments do the majority of sexually abused children of different ages actually receive in terms of amount and type, and which children get it?

The findings

The key question for those planning interventions with sexually abused children and their families is whether psychological treatment can provide benefit or not. We have undertaken a thorough review of the evidence on this question, from which we now extract the principal findings here.*

Through our detailed search of the literature we have been able to find and appraise 14 papers based on seven randomised controlled trials,[12,17,59–65] and four controlled clinical trials.[66–69] This is a limited number as this is a field where high quality research is infrequently conducted.

Here, we provide an overview of the findings and highlight a number of key issues which have implications for practice, with respect to both social care and mental health work.

General points

Time or treatment effects?

In the large majority of studies children's symptoms of distress and psychological disturbance decrease following treatment. These findings apply across a number of the different kinds of treatments that are commonly in use, including group therapy, individual treatment and behavioural treatment.

Two studies suggested that the improvement was due to time passing rather than the effect of specific psychological treatments.[70,71] However, this possibility has been put to the test in a number of studies, with the results strongly suggesting that there is a genuine treatment effect rather than just the passage of time alone.[62,64] These findings are made even more significant because this treatment effect has been shown in studies using different types of therapy; hence we can be reasonably confident that the treatment effects are genuine.

Which symptoms and behaviours are responsive to treatments?

Some behavioural sequelae of sexual abuse have appeared more resistant to treatment efforts than others. Aggression

---

*Details about the full review are available from us, at The Park Hospital for Children, Old Road, Headington, Oxford OX3 7LQ.

and conduct problems, including interpersonal sexual behaviour difficulties, appear to be the most resistant to change.
In some studies, psychological treatment appeared to make
little, if any, impact on these symptoms. On the other hand,
anxiety-related symptoms and depression and feelings of self-
blame did improve in most studies, but not all. There have
been encouraging results from two relatively large-scale
recent studies which have employed cognitive behavioural
treatments specifically focused on the difficulties which
sexually abused children frequently display.[62,64] In these
studies there were reductions in aggressive behaviour and
interpersonal sexual behaviour problems among children.

Which children benefit?

Not all children benefit from therapy, some even get worse,[60]
so a key issue to be addressed is who to offer therapy to.
Although most children and families improve over the time
that they are in a treatment trial, those studies which were
able to demonstrate that their treatment programme was particularly effective were characterised by the fact that they only
treated children who were symptomatic – usually with post-
traumatic stress disorder (PTSD) symptoms.[33,64] So, treatment can be shown to be effective when it is offered to those
children and families with symptoms (of PTSD, or depression, etc.). We discuss this further in the Comment section
below.

As we have already stressed, sexually abused children are
not a homogenous group. Although suffering from one type
of assault, this occurs in a wide range of different psychosocial
contexts and, not surprisingly, results in a variety of possible
outcomes psychologically, including being apparently unaf-
fected. Thus, it is unlikely that one particular form of treatment would cover the needs of all children, especially when
considering the different developmental needs of children of
different ages. Some of the treatment programmes which
have been researched have taken this into account,[12] others
have addressed this problem by examining the effect of treat-

ment in one particular age band[33] or have selectively looked at the effects of treatment among sexually abused children with particular groupings of symptoms.[64] Parents have been included in the therapy 'package' in trials concerned particularly with pre-school children,[33] as well as slightly older (7–13 years) children.[61,64] All of these trials examined a cognitive-behaviour based intervention, with the main difference seeming to be the focus on the different types of symptoms occurring in the different age groups.

There is less evidence to help when issues specific to minority groups or those from socially disadvantaged backgrounds are being considered. One of the research projects we appraised was particularly focused on children with a hearing deficit, and the psychotherapy treatment was modified to take account of this.[69] The group of adolescents who received this therapy did show improvements in their behaviour, but the methodological design of this particular study limits the weight we can place on these findings. A different project from the United States examined a therapy programme designed particularly for the needs of the Afro-American children receiving it.[61] Unfortunately, this was the only one of the trials which specifically took into account the needs of a different (non-Caucasian) ethnic group. Another aspect of concern relates to the study of pre-school children discussed previously.[33] The participants who dropped out from this study tended to be of lower socio-economic class than those who completed the therapy. Although there are several possible reasons for this, it is possible that the therapy was not adapted or explained sufficiently to be made suitable for all the participants.

Importance of supporting the parents (to help the child)

We have already discussed the problems of parents having unmet needs in the child protection arena. Many of the treatment trials have involved at least one non-abusing parent in the therapy – as family network therapy,[12] via a supportive role,[17] or in the individual therapy sessions with the child.[33,61,64] An important finding is that parental support is the strongest family predictor of good outcome for the child,[63] and that involving a (non-abusing) parent in the therapy with the child can help with parents' own problems,[12] as well as leading to them improving their parenting skills and being better able to support their child.[61,64]

As well as involving the parent in the therapy, supporting them outside the treatment is another way of enabling them to support their child better, and this is likely to be a key role for the social worker involved in any case. Two of the research projects ensured that there was a social worker offering continuing support to the parent(s) or carer(s) while the child was in individual or group therapy,[12,17] as they recognised that therapy was far more likely to be successful if stable support outside the therapy was forthcoming. Social work support of the child is also an important element of a treatment package. In the Tavistock therapy trial,[17] social workers were crucial in supporting the child between therapy sessions, and ensuring that the child was able physically to get to the sessions in the first place.

But can everyone use this therapy?

A major issue is the question of whether the psychological treatments which have been studied are of the kind that could be provided in most localities, or whether they are only available in specialised centres and therefore only available to the few rather than the many. Recent research, particularly in the United States, has gone to great lengths to ensure the treatment offered is of a kind that could be duplicated relatively easily.[60,62,64]

Issues of engagement

Treatment drop-out, refusal to engage in treatment or assist their children, or simple denial that there are any problems that need therapeutic help are major issues in all areas of child maltreatment work. It is also the case in sexual abuse that even in those circumstances where children and families initially agree to participate, the therapy programme has to make extensive efforts to ensure subsequent compliance and attendance. Very few of the studies provide us with much detail about which children and families are more likely to drop out, let alone providing an insight into the possible explanations for it. There are many possibilities including the convenience of treatment, accessibility, transport issues, timing, availability of facilities for other younger children, clashes with the school day as well as parental lack of appreciation of the need for or value of psychological treatment. Nonetheless, the lack of treatment and support services is often cited as a major concern of, and complaint by, children and the non-abusive parent.[14]

Can therapy make things worse?

We have so far focused on whether children improve. However, a number of studies report a minority of children who get worse during treatment. This is a very important finding, and may be under-reported in the research which has been conducted to date. Thus, despite receiving treatment there is a group of children who deteriorate, by becoming more anxious, showing greater numbers of post-traumatic fears, or showing more disturbed externalising and aggressive behaviour, combined with the sexual behaviour problems referred to above. Although the numbers will vary, depending on the symptom, the treatment and related factors, it would appear that symptoms actually worsen during the course of treatment in a significant minority.[17]

However, in one study where a significant proportion deteriorated during the year following recognition of sexual abuse,[14] the vast majority of children had not received any specific psychological treatment. Thus, while a minority of children will show an increasing number of symptoms of psychological distress during the one to two years following investigation it is possible that psychological treatment reduces the number and severity. We do not have further data on this issue because the comparative studies have not, for ethical reasons, tended to compare treatment with no treatment but rather one kind of treatment with another.

Which types of psychological treatments work best?

There have been four studies which have looked at the efficacy of group therapy. Two compared it with a form of individual therapy,[17,59] one compared two different forms of group therapy,[60] and one added it to family network treatment.[12] Overall, there seems to be little difference in effect between group and individual treatments in terms of improving symptoms for the child. One of the studies is still being completed,[17] although the results so far suggest that most children improve in both groups over two years.

The most effective treatment (from the available evidence) seems to be short-term focused treatment – of a cognitive-behaviour type.[33,64] When offered to children (from ages 3 to 13) and their parents, there is an improvement in the child's behaviour, including (in younger children at least) in sexualised behaviour and, to a lesser extent, mood. One of the studies compared this cognitive-behaviour therapy with a supportive form of therapy and found the cognitive-behaviour therapy to be far superior. Although there are still only a few treatment trials to support this, the cognitive-behaviour therapies seem more effective in improving children's symptoms than any other form of treatment that has been researched.

These cognitive-behaviour based therapies are described in detail in other publications,[72,73] but the key aim is to target those symptoms commonly experienced by children who have been sexually abused, particularly sadness, aggression, regressive behaviours and sexually inappropriate behaviours in younger children, and abuse-related avoidance and anxiety in older children. A variety of cognitive-behaviour methods can be used to reduce the intensity and frequency of these symptoms, including education, modelling, and body safety skills;[64] however, in older children gradual exposure is the key technique used. This involves encouraging children to confront gradually abuse-related thoughts or situations in a safe environment with the therapist, with the aim of diminishing avoidance and anxiety. Where parents are also involved in the therapeutic programme they are taught about post-traumatic stress disorder (PTSD) symptoms, and helped to respond therapeutically to their child, aiding them in reducing the same fears and avoidance.

Comment

Psychological treatment is associated with improvement for the majority of children, and this finding (derived from controlled trials) is echoed by studies of other designs, examining the rates of improvement in children over time.[74] These show that the improvement with psychological treatment is greater than the improvement with time alone. However, an important minority, perhaps up to 25%, do deteriorate.[48] Symptoms continue unchanged in another group, and a significant number of drop-outs occur. We know relatively little about children and families who either will not attend or drop out prematurely from the treatment. The involvement of the non-abusing parent/child's caretaker is an important aspect of treatment initiatives. Furthermore, we can say that symptomatic children, in particular, do improve in response to psychological treatments. However, this effect may be a consequence of the outcome measures which are used and the length of follow-up utilised in most of the studies. Clearly, if children are not displaying symptoms, symptom checklist-type outcome measures would be unlikely to demonstrate change due to treatment. For these children more subtle measures of mental health and adjustment would be required.

There are many arguments in the field as to whether asymptomatic children should receive treatment. Based on the evidence it is probable they do not require the types of treatment that children with overt symptoms, such as anxiety or depression, will require. The evidence points to the need for treatment to be focused on the symptomatic and to provide them and their carers with help to alleviate problematic symptoms. Work on the coping strategies of relatively resilient children who have been sexually abused lends support to this assertion.[35] In this study, parental support for the child marked out the children who did relatively better. There was an important link, though, between this support and the attributions of the child concerning their own abuse. Thus in this study, at any rate, the children's likelihood of developing healthier attributions about their experience of having been abused was in itself linked to the quality of the parental support that they enjoyed.

Effective treatments have been addressed to the sexual abuse itself, as well as alleviating psychological symptoms. This 'abuse-specific' aspect of the treatment approach includes assisting children to express themselves about sexual abuse, helping them to understand better their experience and unravelling common dynamics involved in sexual abuse.[75] The studies cannot help us decide which elements of abuse-specific treatment are essential: the cathartic unburdening, the unravelling of confusing thoughts about abuse, providing information or addressing symptoms which are common among sexually abused children, such as sleep disturbance. Perhaps it is a combination of all. However, there is good support from the studies for the view that treatment needs to address the particular experience of sexual abuse, and that mere supportive or non-directive treatment is not so effective. There may be some children, however, whose manner of coping has been through denial of experience, where the abuse-specific approach will require adapting and the child's method of managing their distress respected, while trust is gained and their safety assured. Abuse-specific treatments do need to be developmentally sensitive, as well as taking into account issues of disability and race, if they are to be effective for the disparate group of children who comprise the sexually abused.

Professionals sometimes forget that psychological treatment work occurs so often within a context of fear and insecurity for the child. The process of psychological change is intimately bound up with issues to do with their personal safety, and the influence of disturbed and frightening family environments, as well as the child's social and relationship difficulties. Thus, psychological treatment in the field of sexual abuse not only requires adaptation, but also requires that the treatment work is fully integrated with more broadly directed social casework. While, of course, the first priority of such casework will be to make sure the child is safe, it will also be necessary to work on any aspects of the family environment which are disturbed. Other specialists, perhaps working with adult substance abuse or learning disabilities, will be drawn into the net of intervention services surrounding a particular child and family. This is one of the issues which makes the study of outcome in this field a particularly difficult one.

We do not have reliable data on availability, referral patterns or use and take-up of treatment across the United Kingdom. However, what data there are suggest that treatment services are not distributed equitably across the country. It is likely that many factors are involved in the access and use of treatment services. In the first place, children who have been sexually abused tend to be referred for treatment services with higher frequency than children maltreated in other ways. Beyond this finding, it appears that there is substantial variation, geographically, in the availability of treatment services for sexually abused children. There is wide variation in the United Kingdom with respect to the approach of child and adolescent mental health services to accepting referrals of this patient group. Specialised services tend to be located in main university towns and the capital. However, other factors enter the picture. There is variation in social workers' knowledge about local resources and the availability of treatment. It is quite possible that some social workers and general practitioners are relatively more pro-active on behalf of their patients and clients than others. There has been relatively little systematic study of attitudes of referers and the use of local resources. A study in the United States found that ethnicity, having a telephone, and the attitude of the child's mother towards treatment were associated with whether the child and family attended the first therapy appointment.[76] Tingus *et al.*[77] found that children with certain characteristics were more likely to be referred to, or enter, therapy for psychological treatment, as follows: Caucasian children, those of school age, children in 'out of home' placements, or who had been involved with the Criminal Justice System, or the child protection system, and those who had been abused more frequently.

One of the significant limitations of examining randomised controlled trials is they normally only provide evidence about the more specialised or detailed therapies. These in themselves often require special training, although more recent studies from the United States are using therapies which can be more easily learnt and used.[74,78] In addition, there is relatively little attention paid to the surrounding contextual work and supportive work necessary to enable a specific psychological treatment to be effective. For example, there have been few, if any, studies about routine or direct social work with children and families in these situations. Yet the likelihood is, from the results of the studies described, that there is a considerable place for direct work undertaken by social work practitioners, who can provide a major source of support for both children and parents, and carers. They also have a significant role in supporting family members to attend and engage in treatment work.

How then might we assimilate these findings, and apply them within a locality? Perhaps all children who have been sexually abused require some basic education concerning sexuality, sexual roles, and the dynamics of abuse and maltreatment, adapted to their age and developmental status, regardless of whether they are symptomatic or not. Such work could be undertaken by social workers using groups within a relatively brief number of sessions. This would be destigmatising,[79] and would have the added advantage of overcoming the tendency of such children to social isolation.[17] Symptomatic children could be identified and more focused, and if necessary, specialised interventions and plans made for them. In some areas of the country social work practitioners have received specialised training enabling them to work with symptomatic children using a range of psychological treatments. This has the additional advantage of encouraging better links with mental health professionals.

Although there is considerable support for cognitive-behaviour types of intervention for the symptomatic children it would appear that many forms of focused therapy, including group and individual, and family network treatment have some level of support from the studies that have been conducted. Some children will have persistent symptoms of psychological distress which will need specialised treatment focused upon their needs. As has been stressed in this book so far, sexual abuse is a risk factor which can lead to a wide variety of psychological symptoms of disturbance. The evidence from the research studies points towards the need for treatment that focuses on these areas of psychological difficulty and disturbance, while at the same time providing treatment which is sensitive and responsive to the particular problems and dynamics of sexual abuse. Not only that, the treatment will need to be integrated with other systems and professionals who have a legitimate concern with the fact that a child has been sexually exploited[80] (i.e. effective inter-agency working and integration).

There may well be a minority of children who derive benefit from longer term therapy, perhaps of a psychodynamic nature. As yet there are no reliable predictors of who would benefit from this form of treatment,[48] though the use and discussion of its potential use is supplied by Friedrich.[81] Many children are directed towards long-term individual psychodynamic therapy when all else fails, although for such children, short-term focused work of the kind outlined above has usually not been tried in the early stages.

A possible treatment schema is given in Figure 4.

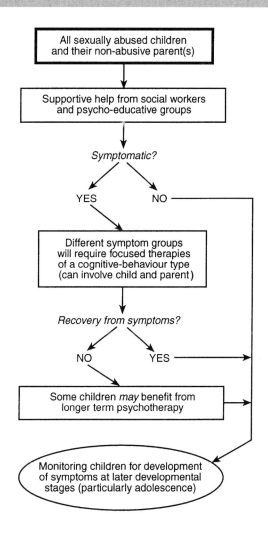

Figure 4 A suggested algorithm for the sexually abused child.

The quality of the helping alliance between practitioners and their patients or clients has been a much neglected area of research in this field, yet is probably crucial when working with families where there has been sexual abuse.[82,83] In a study which did explore the view of children and their parents concerning therapy and intervention, children who had had positive experiences of being in treatment described therapists in terms of their sensitivity, understanding and the concern which they showed for them.[42] However, there were a group of children who described therapy in more negative terms, relaying that it had been difficult for them because they were apparently required to talk about abuse experiences. We do not know whether such children would respond positively to a different type of therapeutic approach. There is, however, a helpful literature concerning the alliance between therapist and client in the field of psychotherapy outcome research generally, as well as among client groups who are particularly difficult to work with.[82,83]

It is vitally important to know *how* the children and their parents show improvements, or indeed deteriorate, during therapy and intervention. At this point, there are some useful leads on this question but no firm data. The likelihood is that therapy for children who have been sexually abused operates via the children's attributions and manner of coping with the trauma which they have suffered. This in turn depends upon their way of thinking and responding to feelings about the abuse; the support, hope and encouragement that they receive from those who care for them, combined with the effective management of behaviour difficulties that they display.

Underpinning everything is the need for the child to be safe from further abuse and to remain safe over subsequent months and years. Hence, it is probable that psychological treatment *per se* will be ineffective without good quality parental care and consistent messages from the social case worker aimed towards these very attributions and opportunities for positive parental support. This places psychological treatment in perspective, for it is our contention that it is of little value alone, unless embedded within good parental care and direct casework. For many children, however, not only is psychological treatment unavailable but they also experience unsafe and inadequate parental care. The added move away from direct social casework towards case management and the focus on the orchestration of services rather than their direct provision represents another lost opportunity to respond to the plight of sexually abused children.

Practice implications

Psychological treatments are more effective than the passage of time alone.

Treatments cannot work in isolation, but require direct social casework support to enable them to be effective, and need to be fully integrated with wider case management.

Children must remain safe from further maltreatment in order to benefit from treatment.

All child victims could benefit from education concerning sexual abuse and its causes and effects, but this would need to be sensitive to the developmental stage of the child.

Symptomatic children can, in addition, benefit from focused treatments.

Of these focused treatments, cognitive-behaviour therapy has the greatest proven benefit for sexually abused children.

Treatments must involve the non-abusive parent or carer.

A variety of treatment approaches need to be available to cover the disparate needs of this population group.

Measuring outcome

Why measure outcome at all?

Research evidence suggests that practitioners often tend to be overoptimistic about outcomes for their clients.[12] So there is a need to have some 'objective' measurements for a number of reasons:

1 to know which treatments/therapies are effective for the child's and family's sake

2 to monitor progress

3 to assist in assessment, and so better understand the needs of the child and family

4 to help decide who and when to refer for more specialised treatment.

Of course, these measures are not a replacement for a good assessment interview and they only cover specific areas of psychological and other functioning, but they can complement a comprehensive assessment, and should be incorporated into everyday practice.

Which measures are useful?

Although we do not aim to provide an exhaustive list, the following measures are helpful because they:

- have generally been well validated
- are checklists and so are quick and easy to use

- have been widely used in research projects, and so enable us
  to compare our clients with those from elsewhere.

Most of the measures cover an aspect of a child's, parent's
or family's functioning, so there is advantage in using
several measures together. The shorter measures are generally more acceptable to clients if several are to be used.
Most of these checklist measures do not require special
training for their administration as they are self-administered
checklist-type questionnaires. However, care should be taken
in the interpretation of results, and they should not be used
as a substitute for a comprehensive assessment and consultation with professionals from other disciplines where this is
appropriate.

We would suggest the use of a general behaviour measure,
a measure of a child's mood, and of sexual behaviour
problems (because of the commonness of depression and
sexualised behaviour problems in sexually abused children).
In addition, some form of assessment of parental mental
health may well be useful. Our choice would be to use a
combination of the Strengths and Difficulties Questionnaire
(for child behaviour), the Child Depression Inventory (for
mood symptoms), the Child Sexual Behaviour Inventory
(for sexualised behaviours) and the General Health Questionnaire (for parents' mood and functioning), as they are relatively short and easy measures to use. However, this is only
a suggestion, and other measures can be helpful. They are
listed below, together with some of the other measures used
in the research.

Measures of child behaviour and emotional state

Strengths and Difficulties Questionnaire[84]

This 25-item questionnaire takes about 5–10 minutes to
complete, and covers a range of problems (emotional,
conduct, peer problems and hyperactivity), as well as
strengths in the form of prosocial behaviour.

Child Behaviour Checklist (CBCL)[85]

A widely used instrument for measuring children's behaviour. There are versions for either parents and teachers to complete for children aged 4–14. It gives a variety of scores covering different areas of functioning (e.g. aggressive, obsessive, hyperactive, somatic) as well as a total behaviour problem score. However, it can take 40 minutes to fill in.

Measures of specific problem areas for children

Child Sexual Behaviour Inventory (CSBI)[32]

A 35-item inventory of sexual behaviours, completed by parents, taking about 15 minutes. It assesses the range and frequency of sexual behaviours in children aged 2–12. The behaviours range from normal sexual behaviour to explicit sexual activity.

Childhood Depression Inventory (CDI)[86]

A 27-item self-report measure that can assess mood-related symptoms in children aged 7–17. It takes 5–10 minutes to complete.

Children's Impact of Traumatic Events Scale – Revised (CITES-R)[87]

A 77-item self-report measure completed by the child. It assesses post-traumatic stress disorder (PTSD) symptoms and trauma-related beliefs.

Measures of parental mental health

General Health Questionnaire (GHQ)[88]

A widely used screening checklist filled in by the parent themselves. The shortest form of this questionnaire has 12 questions. It takes 5–10 minutes to complete.

Beck Depression Inventory (BDI)[89]

> A brief checklist measure completed by the adult about themselves in a few minutes. It gives a rough assessment of whether a parent is depressed or not.

Measures of parent's social support and support for their child

Parenting Practices Questionnaire (PPQ)[90]

> A self-report measure, completed by the parent, which gives an indication of their parenting skills and behaviour.

Parental Reaction to Abuse Disclosure Scale (PRADS)[91]

> This scale is scored by the interviewer after speaking to the mother and child. It has four domains, and takes up to 5 minutes to complete. It assesses a mother's support for the child.

Chapter 11

Conclusions

The following are our current conclusions and recommendations, based upon the best evidence available to us at the time of writing. They may well be able to be changed and refined when further published evidence becomes available.

1 Sexual abuse often occurs against a background of other family problems, and is linked with other forms of abuse (physical, emotional and neglect).

2 The abused child's parents, especially the non-abusive caretaker, face major stress and may have considerable psychological needs, particularly during the beginning of a complicated and often stressful professional investigation of concerns about sexual abuse. Parents' needs are frequently rendered secondary and there is evidence that parental needs prove difficult for professionals to appreciate fully. However, meeting the needs of, and involving, the non-abusing parent in investigation and intervention is associated with a better outcome for the child. Hence, although there are considerable difficulties in working in partnership with some parents, it would appear to be a particularly fruitful focus for professional involvement.

3 The approach and style of the initial contact appears crucial to engagement and the ability to work with families.

4 Abused children and their parents often have psychological problems related to or as a consequence of the

abuse. Whilst protection from further abuse is obviously the first essential task in responding to abuse, these psychological problems are often inadequately addressed when assessing and planning an intervention with the child and family. This conclusion is as applicable to extra-familial sexual abuse as intra-familial.

5   Intervention can be, and often is effective. Protecting the child, increasing the social support available to the child and their family, and treating psychological symptoms and behaviours associated with abuse can be done, although it is unlikely that all these aims could be achieved by one single worker. A team, or core group approach, and greater cross-disciplinary working with mental health professionals are likely to be better suited to meeting the many and varied needs of children and families in this predicament.

6   Some therapies are effective in helping children cope with symptoms of depression, anxiety and post-traumatic stress disorder, and with sexualised and other behavioural problems. They can also improve the outcome for parents when they are involved, which in turn leads to greater benefit for their child. Support for the child and family outside of the therapy sessions will also usually improve outcome.

7   The best available evidence points to the use of focused therapies based on a cognitive-behaviour model being the most effective way of treating these symptoms. This is most effective when a parent is also included in the programme. Non-directive supportive and psychodynamic therapies lack empirical support at present. Group therapy compares favourably with these individual supportive therapies.

8   No single therapy has demonstrable benefit for all children who have been sexually abused, and whilst it makes sense to commend those therapies (such as cognitive-behaviour therapy), which are undoubtedly effective in some circum-

stances, one implication from the treatment outcome studies is that flexibility within treatment programmes, or alternatively a range of available treatments, is absolutely essential if the variety of psychological outcomes and consequences of sexual abuse are to be addressed in therapy, as well as the broad variety of ages and special needs of the child victims. There are no studies on children with learning disabilities, and studies demonstrating developmentally sensitive treatments are still required.

9 Substitute care can expose children to increased risk, and it is essential that the needs of children in substitute care are regularly monitored. They often fall through the net in terms of receiving treatment and appropriate support once placed in care.

10 There are currently inadequate efforts made to monitor the effectiveness of interventions for children and their families where a child has been sexually abused. Appropriate therapeutic help is rarely offered, and cases are often closed with many outstanding needs remaining for the child and family. Objective measures of outcome are rarely used, so unhelpful therapies continue to be offered.

Chapter 12

Implications for practitioners

Practitioners will doubtless refer to the practice implications of each chapter, and then back to the findings and comments sections, in order to draw out points important for their everyday practice. We think the research itself, summarised and cited in Appendix B, will be a useful resource to illuminate specific areas of practice. That said, the following prominent themes emerge from the research.

1 Child sexual abuse occurs within the context of a range of other difficulties for the child and her/his family. This necessitates a breadth of assessment and intervention services. Assessment approaches which are informed by a developmental and ecological perspective (*see* page 2) are the most likely ones to encompass this broad range of needs.[47]

2 Integration of professional inputs at all stages – assessment, as well as planning and delivering interventions – is essential in order to achieve desirable outcomes. These outcomes incorporate keeping the child safe, ensuring or improving general caretaking and parenting, treating symptoms of psychological disorder in children and/or adults, and containing sexually aggressive, violent, or exploitative behaviour. The professional inputs incorporate child protection work, direct social work and support, psychological treatments, child health surveillance and 'psychoeducation'.

3 The needs of the child and caretaker or parent change over time, requiring continuing assessments/case planning,

rather than single assessments of risk. Only in this way will the sleeper effects of sexual abuse be discovered, and appropriate help offered. Discharging children and families once the immediate issues of protection have been dealt with is an inadequate response, even if it is understandable given the pressures under which practitioners sometimes operate.

4 Understanding the perspectives of children and parents/ carers is crucial if effective partnership is to be achieved. Partnership may not always be feasible, or safe so far as the child is concerned. However, parents can better tolerate and appreciate the nature of the professional intervention, even if unwelcome or stressful, if they are kept informed as to its purpose, and can understand what professionals are trying to achieve.

5 Intervention implies a range of different activities if the breadth of problems which the child and/or family have are to be adequately addressed. These include direct social casework, assuring the child's safety and protection, education for children and families, support through the crisis which follows discovery of sexual abuse, and psychological treatments. Intervention plans need to be linked to hoped-for outcomes and associated with time scales which are developmentally appropriate to the child's needs, as well as practically achievable.

6 Practitioners need appropriate supervision and support in order to be able to function safely and to a high standard in this area.

7 Certain groups of children who have been sexually abused require particular mention because they frequently receive fewer services than they require. These are children abused by persons outside the immediate household (extra-familial abuse), and those children in substitute care.

8 Psychological treatments are effective with sexually abused children and their families. These treatments need to be

embedded and integrated with broader social casework, but nonetheless can contribute to improved outcomes for this group of children and their families. Persistent psychological symptoms occur in a significant minority of children, and for these a range of other treatment approaches may need to be available to try and help them, because the outcome for this group is poor if their psychological distress and sequelae remain untreated.

Implications for managers and supervisors of practitioners

Supervisors, senior practitioners, and those who manage small groups of front-line practitioners vary in the extent to which they continue with direct work with children and families. Hence, many of the implications of the previous section are relevant to managers, too. However, we feel the following themes derive from the research findings, and may be particularly helpful. The supervisory role is key to ensuring a high quality of assessment, case planning and intervention, frequently within a climate of resource constraint, while maintaining the focus of the team on the desired outcome for children and families.

1 Support and supervision of front-line workers is crucial to effective, good quality work with sexually abused children and their families.

2 Sufficient time is needed for planning purposes, both strategic planning prior to initial contact and interviewing as well as planning with other agencies and professionals in the aftermath of case registration.

3 Children who have been sexually abused, together with their families, present a wide variety of needs, including those deriving from the sexual assault itself, but also extending to a range of other problems affecting the child and family members. These needs may change during the life of a case, requiring continuing assessment and varia-

tions in the response of services. A narrow child protection focus can obscure the broader needs of sexually abused children and their families.

4 Although partnership is desirable and achievable with many children and family members it may not be possible at all stages in the process of investigation and intervention. In some circumstances the focus on partnership would need to give way to the child's more pressing welfare.

5 There is a major role for direct work from social workers, providing psychosocial support and essential education for children and mothers, as well as providing continuing direct work for these families. Additional training for front-line social workers would add significantly to the resources which a children and families social work team could provide. This is likely to enhance morale within social work teams.

6 It will be necessary to establish good working links, and policies between different professionals, agencies and the relevant specialist personnel. Examples include children with disability, children and young people with severe psychiatric problems, and those with language and communication difficulties.

7 There are subgroups of cases where, even if child protection is achieved, significant needs remain unmet. These include those children who are in substitute care, whose needs for direct work, support and psychological treatments appear to be frequently unmet, as well as those who are abused by persons besides their parents or immediate carers.

8 Interpersonal sexual behaviour problems among sexually abused children present a significant challenge to children and family services. However, their needs for therapeutic intervention span many of the requirements of those who do not display such problems. This group are important because they represent a significant minority of sexually abused children.[30]

9 Major training implications flow from the findings on assessment and intervention. Training will need to be made available in order to assure consistent quality by all staff working in children and families teams, but particularly for those working in this stressful field.

Implications for planners and commissioners of services

Good quality intervention services do result in demonstrable benefit for sexually abused children and their parents or carers. Given the long-term ill effects of child sexual abuse, they are therefore a good investment. There are significant opportunities to prevent cycles of future child maltreatment and parenting difficulties, which make intervention with this group of children and families a major priority. Interventions are likely to play a significant role in achieving the important outcome of social inclusion for this population, both in the short and long term. These comments apply especially to the subgroup of children who are placed in substitute care who currently have significantly poor outcomes in terms of mental health, social adjustment, education and future employment opportunities.

1 A broad range of services is required in order to meet the disparate needs of this population group. At the same time there needs to be a move towards offering interventions and treatments which are shown to be effective and evidence based, in particular the cognitive-behaviour based therapies for symptomatic children. In non-symptomatic sexually abused children, group psychoeducational sessions could be offered, particularly as they are both as effective and cheaper than individual, non-directive, and psychodynamic therapies. More expensive therapies should be retained within the broad portfolio of services available within an area, including the need for residential and in-patient psychiatric treatments for a minority of children and young people.

2 The refocusing of children's services and the enhancement of supportive services for children and families should not lead to a dismantling of the all-important protection services. Findings from this research on the numbers of children remaining unsafe and vulnerable despite intervention emphasise this point.

3 Procedures and explicit policies for assessment, planning and intervention are vital for each area. Nonetheless, it must be acknowledged that many children and families do not proceed along a linear path and the trajectory of many cases is atypical. Hence, the research findings argue for an emphasis upon the quality of services at the point of delivery, within a broad procedural framework, rather than a focus on audit and review of procedure alone.

4 Work in the field of child sexual abuse is highly stressful for all professionals involved, hence the need for effective and sufficient supervision and support for staff. The research emphasises that this is a necessity rather than merely a desirable feature of services.

5 Training will be necessary for the effective delivery of assessment, planning and treatment services with this client group. It is likely to prove a good investment, given the support for the interventions outlined in this report, as well as the likely implications of preventing cycles of parenting difficulty and child maltreatment in future generations.

6 The above considerations raise significant challenges for the encouragement of locally sensitive solutions on the one hand versus fundamental fairness and equity of services on an area or national basis on the other. In view of the significant negative effects which flow from inadequate provision, we think the case for achieving a basic level of equitable services, of the kind implied by these research findings, is overwhelming.

7 Achieving the necessary integration of the different agency and professional contributions responding to child sexual abuse brings with it significant problems for overcoming boundaries and the traditional territories of the professions involved. Whilst this is undoubtedly the case for a wide range of problems affecting children, it is brought into relief by the research findings in this particular area.

8 There is a need for greater integration and closer links between social work and health, as well as other professions and agencies, because currently the needs of these children and their families are not being adequately addressed, dealt with or responded to. Such integration does not imply a merging of professional roles and responsibilities; on the contrary, it would depend on retaining and sharpening the focus and identity of different professional inputs.

9 Greater integration within health services is also required, in particular overcoming problems of the interface between adult and child mental health services.

10 The role of Area Child Protection Committees (ACPCs) is fundamental to attaining the objectives which are implied above. ACPCs are well-established forums which effectively integrate the activities of numerous professionals and agencies around the central objective of responding to child protection concerns. In addition, appropriate mechanisms will be needed to link the activities of ACPCs to the wider picture of children's services planning.

References

1 National Research Council (Panel on research into child abuse and neglect) (1993) Etiology of child maltreatment. In: *Understanding Child Abuse and Neglect*, pp 106–60. National Academy Press, Washington DC.

2 Jones DPH (1997) Treatment of the child and the family where child abuse or neglect has occurred. In: R Helfer, R Kempe and R Krugman (eds) *The Battered Child* (5th edn), pp 521–542. University of Chicago Press, Chicago.

3 Belsky J (1980) Child maltreatment: an ecological integration. *American Psychologist*. **35**: 320–35.

4 Cicchetti D (1989) How research on child maltreatment has informed the study of child development: perspectives from developmental psychopathology. In: D Cicchetti and V Carlson (eds) *Child Maltreatment: theory and research on the causes and consequences of child abuse and neglect*, pp 377–431. Cambridge University Press, Cambridge.

5 Belsky J (1993) Etiology of child maltreatment: a developmental/ecological analysis. *Psychological Bulletin*. **114**: 413–34.

6 Birchall E and Hallett C (1995) *Working Together in Child Protection*. HMSO, London.

7 Calam R, Cox A, Glasgow D, Jimmieson P and Groth Larsen S (1999) *The Development of a Computer Assisted Interview for Children*. (Report submitted to the Department of Health.)

8 Cleaver H and Freeman P (1995) *Parental Perspectives in Cases of Suspected Child Abuse*. HMSO, London.

9 Farmer E and Owen M (1995) *Child Protection Practice: private risks and public remedies*. HMSO, London.

10 Farmer E and Pollock S (1998) *Sexually Abused and Abusing Children in Substitute Care*. Wiley, Chichester.

11 Hallett C (1995) *Inter-agency Co-ordination in Child Protection*. HMSO, London.

12 Monck E, Bentovim A, Goodall G, Hyde C, Lwin R, Sharland E and Elton A (1996) *Child Sexual Abuse: a descriptive and treatment study*. HMSO, London.

13 Monck E and New M (1996) *Sexually Abused Children and Adolescents and Young Perpetrators of Sexual Abuse who were Treated in Voluntary Community Facilities*. HMSO, London.

14 Sharland E, Seal H, Croucher M, Aldgate J and Jones D (1996) *Professional Intervention in Child Sexual Abuse*. HMSO, London.

15 Skuse D, Bentovim A, Hodges J, Stevenson J, Andreou C, Lanyado M, Williams B, New M and McMillan D (1998) *The Influence of Early Experience of Sexual Abuse on the Formation of Sexual Preferences during Adolescence*. (Report submitted to the Department of Health.)

16 Skuse D, Bentovim A, Hodges J, Stevenson J, Andreou C, Lanyado M, New M, Williams B and McMillan D (1998) Risk factors for the development of sexually abusive behaviour in sexually victimised adolescent males: cross sectional study. *British Medical Journal*. **317**: 175–9.

17 Trowell J, Kolvin I, Weeramanthri T, Berelowitz M, Sadowski H, Rushton A, Miles G, Glaser D, Elton A, Rustin M and Hunter M (1998) *Psychotherapy Outcome Study for Sexually Abused Girls*. (Report submitted to the Department of Health).

18 Finkelhor D and Berliner L (1995) Research on the treatment of sexually abused children: a review and recommendations. *Journal of the American Academy of Child and Adolescent Psychiatry*. **34**: 1408–23.

19 Oxford and Anglia R&D Webpage: *http//www.ihs.ox.ac.uk/library/filters.html*

20 Guyatt GH, Sackett DL and Cook DJ (1994) Users' Guides. How to use an article on therapy or prevention. *Journal of the American Medical Association*. **271**: 59–63.

21 McMaster University. *Qualitative Research – quality filters for evidence based journals.* (Personal communication from Dr John Geddes, February 1998)

22 Greenhalgh T (1997) *How to Read a Paper.* BMJ Publishing Group, London.

23 Department of Health (1991*) Working Together under the Children Act, 1989: a guide to arrangements for inter-agency cooperation for the protection of children from abuse.* HMSO, London.

24 Parton N (1997) Child protection and family support: current debates and future prospects. In: N Parton (ed) *Child Protection and Family Support: tensions, contradictions and possibilities,* pp 1–24. Routledge, London.

25 Mullen P, Martin J, Anderson J *et al.* (1993) Childhood sexual abuse and mental health in adult life. *British Journal of Psychiatry.* **163**: 721–32.

26 Madonna P, Van Scoyk S and Jones DPH (1991) Family interactions within incest and non-incest families. *American Journal of Psychiatry.* **148**: 46–9.

27 Furniss T (1991) *The Multiprofessional Handbook of Child Sexual Abuse.* Routledge, London.

28 Bentovim A (1992) *Trauma Organised Systems: physical and sexual abuse in families.* Karnac, London.

29 Van Scoyk S, Gray J and Jones DPH (1988) A theoretical framework for evaluation and treatment of the victims of child sexual assault by a non family member. *Family Process.* **27**: 105–13.

30 Hall DK, Mathews F and Pearce J (1998) Factors associated with sexual behavior problems in young sexually abused children. *Child Abuse and Neglect.* **22**: 1045–63.

31 Jones DPH (1998). Editorial: Sexual behavior problems among sexual abused children. *Child Abuse and Neglect.* **22**: 1043–44.

32 Friedrich WN, Grambsch P, Broughton D, Kuiper J and Beilke RL (1991) Normative sexual behavior in children. *Pediatrics.* **88**: 456–64.

33 Cohen JA and Mannarino AP (1997) A treatment outcome study

for sexually abused preschool children: outcome during a one-year follow-up. *Journal of the American Academy of Child and Adolescent Psychiatry.* **36**: 1228–35.

34 Chaffin M, Wherry J and Dykman R (1996) School aged children's coping with sexual abuse: abuse stresses and symptoms associated with four coping strategies. *Child Abuse and Neglect.* **21**: 227–40.

35 Spaccarelli S and Kim S (1995) Resilience criteria and factors associated with resilience in sexually abused girls. *Child Abuse and Neglect.* **19**: 1171–82.

36 Runtz M and Schallow J (1997) Social support and coping strategy as mediators of adult adjustment following a childhood maltreatment. *Child Abuse and Neglect.* **21**: 211–26.

37 Fonagy P, Leigh T, Steele M, Steele H, Kennedy R, Matton G and Gerber A (1996) The relation of attachment status, psychiatric classification and response to psychotherapy. *Journal of Consulting and Clinical Psychology.* **64**(1): 22–31.

38 Social Services Inspectorate/Department of Health (1994) *The Child, The Court and The Video: a study of the implementation of the memorandum on good practice on video interviewing child witnesses.* Department of Health Publications, Wetherby, Yorks.

39 Department of Health (1995) *Child Protection: messages from research.* HMSO, London.

40 Home Office and Department of Health (1992) *Memorandum of Good Practice on Video Interviewing of Child Witnesses.* Department of Health Publications, Wetherby, Yorks.

41 Gibbons J, Conroy S and Bell C (1995) *Operating the Child Protection System: a study of child protection practices in English local authorities.* HMSO, London.

42 Berliner L and Conte J (1995) The effects of disclosure and intervention on sexually abused children. *Child Abuse and Neglect.* **19**: 371–84.

43 Thoburn J, Lewis A and Shemmings D (1995) *Paternalism or Partnership? Family involvement in the child protection process.* HMSO, London.

44 Henry J (1997) System intervention trauma to child sexual abuse victims following disclosure. *Journal of Interpersonal Violence.* **12**: 499–512.

45 Lask J (1994) Social work in child psychiatry settings. In: M Rutter, E Taylor and L Hersov (eds) *Child and Adolescent Psychiatry: modern approaches*, pp 900–17. Blackwell, Oxford.

46 Social Services Inspectorate, Department of Health (1997) *Messages from Inspection: child protection inspections, 1992–1996*. Department of Health Publications, Wetherby, Yorks.

47 Department of Health (In press) *Framework for Assessing Children and their Families*. The Stationery Office, London.

48 Tebbutt J, Swanston H, Oates RK and O'Toole BI (1997) Five years after child sexual abuse: persisting dysfunction and problems of prediction. *Journal of the American Academy of Child and Adolescent Psychiatry.* **36**: 330–9.

49 Finkelhor D (1994) Current information on the scope and nature of child sexual abuse. *The Future of Children.* **4**: 31–53.

50 Fergusson DM, Lynskey MT and Horwood LJ (1996) Childhood sexual abuse and psychiatric disorder in young adulthood: 1. prevalence of sexual abuse and factors associated with sexual abuse. *Journal of the American Academy of Child and Adolescent Psychiatry.* **35**: 1355–64.

51 Cohen JA and Mannarino AP (1996) Factors that mediate treatment outcome of sexually abused preschool children. *Journal of the American Academy of Child and Adolescent Psychiatry.* **35**: 1402–10.

52 Levy H, Markovic J, Chaudhry U, Ahart S and Torres H (1995) Reabuse rates in a sample of children followed for 5 years after discharge from a child abuse inpatient assessment programme. *Child Abuse and Neglect.* **19**: 1363–77.

53 Dingwall R, Eekelaar J and Murray T (1983) *The Protection of Children: state intervention and family life*. Blackwell, Oxford.

54 Department of Health (1998) *Working Together to Safeguard Children: new government proposals for inter-agency cooperation*. Consultation paper. Department of Health Publications, Wetherby, Yorks.

55　Utting W, Baines C, Stuart M, Rolands J and Vialva R (1997) *People Like Us. The report of the review of the safeguards for children living away from home*. HMSO, London.

56　Davies G, Wilson C, Mitchell R and Milsom J (1995) *Video Taping Children's Evidence: an evaluation*. Home Office, London.

57　Goodman GS, Pyle L, Jones DPH, Port L and Prado L (1992) Testifying in court: emotional effects of criminal court testimony on child sexual assault victims. *Monographs of the Society for Research in Child Development*. **57** (5, Serial No. 229), 1–161.

58　Runyan D, Everson M, Edelsohn G, Hunter W and Coulter M (1988) Impact of legal intervention on sexually abused children. *Journal of Pediatrics*. **113**: 647–53.

59　Baker CR (1987) A comparison of individual and group therapy as treatment of sexually abused adolescent females. *Dissertation Abstracts International*. **47**(10-B): 4319–20.

60　Berliner L and Saunders B (1996) Treating fear and anxiety in sexually abused children: results of a controlled, two year follow-up study. *Child Maltreatment*. **1**: 294–309.

61　Celano M, Hazard A, Webb C and McCall C (1996) Treatment of traumagenic beliefs among sexually abused girls and their mothers: an evaluation study. *Journal of Abnormal Child Psychology*. **24**: 1–17.

62　Cohen JA and Mannarino AP (1996) A treatment outcome study for sexually abused preschool children: Initial findings. *Journal of the American Academy of Child and Adolescent Psychiatry*. **35**: 42–50.

63　Cohen JA and Mannarino AP (1998) Factors that mediate treatment outcome of sexually abused preschool children: six- and 12-month follow-up. *Journal of the American Academy of Child and Adolescent Psychiatry*. **37**: 44–51.

64　Deblinger E, Lippman J and Steer R (1996) Sexually abused children suffering post-traumatic stress symptoms: initial treatment outcome findings. *Child Maltreatment*. **1**: 310–21.

65 Hyde C, Bentovim A and Monck E (1995) Some clinical and methodological implications of a treatment study of sexually abused children. *Child Abuse and Neglect.* **19**: 1387–99.

66 Downing J, Jenkins SJ and Fisher GL (1988) A comparison of psychodynamic and reinforcement treatment with sexually abused children. *Elementary School Guidance and Counselling.* **22**: 291–8.

67 McGain B and McKinzey RK (1995) The efficacy of group treatment in sexually abused girls. *Child Abuse and Neglect.* **19**: 1157–69.

68 Verleur D, Hughes RE and Dobkin de Rios M (1986) Enhancement of self-esteem among female adolescent incest victims: a controlled comparison. *Adolescence.* **84**: 843–54.

69 Sullivan PM, Scanlan JM, Brookhouser PE, Schulte LE and Knutson JF (1992) The effects of psychotherapy on behaviour problems of sexually abused deaf children. *Child Abuse and Neglect.* **16**: 297–307.

70 Gomes Schwartz B, Horowitz J and Cardarelli A (1990) *Child Sexual Abuse: the initial effects.* Sage, London.

71 Oates RK, O'Toole B, Lynch D, Stern A and Cooney G (1994) Stability and change in outcomes for sexually abused children. *Journal of the American Academy of Child and Adolescent Psychiatry.* **33**: 945–53.

72 Deblinger E and Heflin AH (1996) *Treating Sexually Abused Children and their Non-offending Parents: a cognitive behavioural approach.* Sage, London.

73 Cohen J and Mannarino AP (1993) A treatment model for sexually abused pre-schoolers. *Journal of Interpersonal Violence.* **8**: 115–31.

74 Lanktree C and Briere J (1995) Outcome of therapy for sexually abused children: a repeated measures study. *Child Abuse and Neglect.* **19**: 1145–56.

75 Berliner L (1997) Intervention with children who experienced trauma. In: D Cicchetti and S Toth (eds) *Developmental Perspectives on Trauma: theory, research and intervention*, pp 491–514. University of Rochester Press, Rochester, NY.

76 Haskett M, Nowlan N, Hutchesone J and Whitworth J (1991) Factors associated with successful therapy in child sexual abuse cases. *Child Abuse and Neglect.* **15**: 467–76.

77 Tingus K, Heger A, Foy D and Leskin G (1996) Factors associated with entry into therapy in children evaluated for sexual abuse. *Child Abuse and Neglect.* **20**: 63–8.

78 Staufer L and Deblinger E (1996) Cognitive behavioural groups for non-offending mothers and their young sexually abused children: a preliminary treatment outcome study. *Child Maltreatment.* **1**: 65–76.

79 Finkelhor D and Brown A (1985) The traumatic impact of child sexual abuse: a conceptualisation. *American Journal of Orthopsychiatry.* **55**: 530–41.

80 Jones DPH (1996) Management of the sexually abused child. *Advances in Psychiatric Treatment.* **2**: 39–45.

81 Friedrich WN (1990) Individual treatment. In: WN Friedrich (ed.) *Psychotherapy of Sexually Abused Children and their Families*, pp 131–66. Norton, London.

82 Jones DPH (1996) Editorial: The helping alliance in work with families where children have been abused or neglected. *Child Abuse and Neglect.* **20**: 345–7.

83 Morrison-Dore M and Alexander L (1996) The helping alliance. *Child Abuse and Neglect.* **20**: 349–61.

84 Goodman R (1997) The strengths and difficulties questionnaire: a research note. *Journal of Child Psychology and Psychiatry.* **38**: 581–6.

85 Achenbach TM and Edelbrock C (1983) *Manual for the Child Behavior Checklist and Revised Child Behavior Profile.* University of Vermont Department of Psychiatry, Burlington, VT.

86 Kovacs M (1983) *The Children's Depression Inventory: a self-rated depression scale for school-aged youngsters.* University of Pittsburgh School of Medicine, Pittsburgh, PA.

87 Wolfe VV, Gentile C, Michienzi T, Sas L and Wolfe D (1991) The Children's Impact of Traumatic Events Scale: a measure of

post-sexual abuse PTSD symptoms. *Behavioral Assessment*. **13**: 359–83.

88 Goldberg D (1987) *Manual of the General Health Questionnaire*. NFER, Windsor, UK.

89 Beck AT, Steer RA and Garsin MA (1988) Psychometric properties of the Beck Depression Inventory: twenty-five years of evaluation. *Clinical Psychology Review*. **8**: 77–100.

90 Strayhorn JM and Weidman CS (1988) A parental practices scale and its relation to parent and child mental health. *Journal of the American Academy of Child and Adolescent Psychiatry*. **27**: 613–18.

91 Everson M, Hunter W, Runyan D, Edelsohn G and Coulter M (1989) Maternal support following disclosure of incest. *American Journal of Orthopsychiatry*. **59**: 197–207.

92 Brown D and Pedder J (1979) *Introduction to Psychotherapy*. Tavistock, London.

Department of Health funded projects

Birchall E and Hallett C (1995) *Working Together in Child Protection*. HMSO, London.

Calam R, Cox A, Glasgow D, Jimmieson P and Groth Larsen S (1998) *The Development of a Computer Assisted Interview for Children*. Report submitted to Department of Health.

Cleaver H and Freeman P (1995) *Parental Perspectives in Cases of Suspected Child Abuse*. HMSO, London.

Farmer E and Owen M (1995) *Child Protection Practice: private risks and public remedies*. HMSO, London.

Farmer E and Pollock S (1998) *Sexually Abused and Abusing Children in Substitute Care*. Wiley, Chichester.

Hallett C (1995) *Inter-agency Co-ordination in Child Protection*. HMSO, London.

Monck E, Bentovim A, Goodall G, Hyde C, Lwin R, Sharland E and Elton A (1996) *Child Sexual Abuse: a descriptive and treatment study*. HMSO, London.

Monck E and New M (1996) *Sexually Abused Children and Adolescents and Young Perpetrators of Sexual Abuse who were Treated in Voluntary Community Facilities*. HMSO, London.

Sharland E, Seal H, Croucher H, Aldgate J and Jones D (1996) *Professional Intervention in Child Sexual Abuse.* HMSO, London.

Skuse D, Bentovim A, Hodges J, Stevenson J, Andreou C, Lanyado M, Williams B, New M and McMillan D (1998) *The Influence of Early Experience of Sexual Abuse on the Formation of Sexual Preferences during Adolescence.* (Report submitted to the Department of Health.)

Trowell J, Kolvin I, Berelowitz M, Weeramanthri T, Sadowski H, Rushton A, Miles G, Glaser D, Elton A, Rustin M and Hunter M (1998) *Psychotherapy Outcome Study for Sexually Abused Girls.* (Report submitted to the Department of Health.)

Summaries of studies

Birchall E and Hallett C (1995) *Working Together in Child Protection*. HMSO, London

Aim

Exploration of professionals' views of co-ordination in child protection.

Methods

A questionnaire survey of staff groups involved in child protection from three areas in the north of England was undertaken, using a specifically designed questionnaire, with a mix of questions and case vignettes.

A stratified random sample was taken from each of the following professional groups:

Social workers   Health visitors   Teachers
General practitioners   Paediatricians   Police
Local authority lawyers NSPCC workers

Selected key results

339 responses (60% response rate).

Social workers, police, paediatricians and health visitors were the professional groups most involved in the child protection network.

Recording of information by key workers was poor, particularly of communication with other agencies.

Approximately two-thirds thought that co-ordination between professionals worked well in the assessment phase. However, views were more mixed regarding the later stages of child protection work – nearly 75% thought co-ordination worked well, but 25% thought it worked badly.

General practitioners rarely attended case conferences, despite being invited.

Strengths of study

Survey of a large number of practitioners.

Wide range of professionals surveyed, from a range of socio-economic areas.

Stratified random sampling used.

Limitations of study

Some professional groups were over-represented – relatively small numbers of social workers and police were included.

Responses from lawyers were excluded from the study completely, as few of them replied.

Calam R, Cox A, Glasgow D, Jimmieson P and Groth Larsen S (1998) *The Development of a Computer Assisted Interview for Children.* (Unpublished report)

Aim

To develop a computer assisted interview to aid interviewing where abuse is suspected.

Methods

Developed in a modular fashion, through an initial feasibility study, followed by piloting in several different sites and formats.

Although designed for 8- to 12-year-olds, it has been used with children aged 4 years and upwards.

Strengths of design

It can be an enjoyable and novel experience for the child, facilitating discussion with an interviewer, and it is flexible, with a variety of different modules and different languages (including sign language).

May be particularly useful with children where communication is difficult, for example those with learning disability, elective mutism, or attention problems.

Limitations of design

At this stage, the interview has only been piloted in two small studies, so needs wider piloting and use.

Cleaver H and Freeman P (1995) *Parental Perspectives in Cases of Suspected Child Abuse*. HMSO, London.

Aim

To explore parental perspectives in the context of suspected abuse.

Methods

Stage 1 All cases from two local authorities, where abuse (of all types) was seriously considered by police, social workers, health visitors or probation over a one-year period (583 children), were examined.

Stage 2 The cases of 30 families were studied in more detail (about one quarter of the children in these families were considered at risk of sexual abuse). Family members and involved professionals were interviewed, and the families were observed as part of the study.

Selected key results

Abuse often occurs against a background of multiple other problems (e.g. ill-health, unemployment, poor housing).

The perspectives of parents and professionals can often be very different early on in an investigation.

Perspectives on what is happening during the child protection process can, and do change.

Strengths of study

A detailed study using a mix of quantitative and qualitative methods.

Several different sources of information were used – both parents and professionals were interviewed, families were observed by the researchers, and the researchers attended all relevant meetings.

Limitations of study

All types of abuse were considered, not just sexual abuse, so we cannot always assume that the results are truly representative of cases of sexual abuse.

The methods of analysing data were not always made explicit – so there may be some bias, depending on the researchers' perspective.

Farmer E and Owen M (1995) *Child Protection Practice: private risks and public remedies*. HMSO, London.

Aims

To examine consumer views of the child protection process, to explore the interventions routinely offered and to examine the decision-making process and outcomes for children on the Child Protection Register.

Methods

> *Stage 1* The researchers attended 120 child protection confer-ences in three local authorities during 1989–90.

> *Stage 2* Where children were registered (for any form of abuse) at the child protection conference, their families and key workers were interviewed, as were older children. The interviews were carried out soon after registration, with a follow-up interview 20 months later. A semi-structured inter-view was used, including some objective measures such as the Child Depression Inventory and the Malaise scale.

Selected key results

> Family violence was or had been a feature in over half the families.

> It was often mothers or children themselves who brought the abuse to the attention of Social Services, with the expectation that they would receive some help.

> Sexual abuse often occurred in combination with physical abuse and/or neglect.

Strengths of study

> Used a mixture of qualitative and quantitative methods – interviews with several informants, as well as attending the child protection conferences.

> Repeated interviews allowed the researchers to follow the pattern of cases through time.

Limitations of study

> The study only included cases where everyone agreed to be interviewed.

> 26% of the children and families who qualified for Stage 2 of the study refused to take part. This may have lead to some

bias in the sample towards including the more co-operative families.

Farmer E and Pollock S (1998) *Sexually Abused and Abusing Children in Substitute Care*. Wiley, Chichester

Aims

To provide information about the placement of these children in residential and foster care and to examine the way in which they were cared for during their placements.

Methods

Stage 1 The case files of all children newly 'looked after', during the time scale of study (1993–94), from two local authorities were examined (250 case files).

Stage 2 Those who were sexually abused or abusers were interviewed (40 children), as were their caregivers and social workers.

Selected key results

The mix of other children in a placement is often not considered when a placement decision is made – even for a vulnerable group such as sexually abused children.

Many of the sexually abused or abusive children had been placed for reasons other than the sexual abuse.

Sexualised behaviour was seen in many of the children, leading to pregnancy or prostitution in some cases. Little educational work on sexualised behaviour and safety was undertaken with the children, despite these concerns.

Only a minority of the children were offered therapeutic help.

Strengths of study

> A detailed interview was undertaken with the young people and others involved in each case, so several different perspectives were considered.

> The children who were followed included some in an early, and others at a later, stage of their placements.

Limitations of study

> The 40 children interviewed included some children (15) newly looked after in a second time period because insufficient children in the original case file sample met the criteria for Stage 2 of the study.

> The children who were interviewed in Stage 2 were a more troubled group than those who had moved on from substitute care, so they may be unrepresentative of 'looked after' children as a whole.

Hallett C (1995) *Inter-agency Co-ordination in Child Protection*. HMSO, London

Aim

> To explore co-ordination through the whole child protection process.

Methods

> *Stage 1* A random stratified sample of 48 cases, where a child of primary school age had been physically or sexually abused, were selected and the case files reviewed.

> *Stage 2* Eight of these cases were selected by a similar method and interviews conducted with all the key professionals involved. These professionals also completed a questionnaire.

Selected key results

In over half the cases of sexual abuse the referral was made by the child's mother.

At this time, parental attendance at child protection conferences was rare, and the majority of time in the conference was spent on registration, with little time spent on the child protection plan.

The key problems identified in monitoring the implementation of services planned at the conference were:

1 poor recording in social work notes

2 lack of parental co-operation in some cases

3 a change in the case or child circumstances

4 lack of resources

5 lack of ongoing inter-agency work and co-operation.

Strengths of study

A variety of professionals were interviewed in detail.

The study links in with, and complements, previous research projects (*see* Birchall and Hallett, 1995).

Limitations of study

As the study is based on 48 selected cases, the results may be specific to this group in three ways, and so not necessarily applicable to the wider 'abused' population:

1 only cases of physical and sexual abuse were considered

2 only children of primary school age were included (4–11 years)

3 only registered cases of abuse were included.

Monck E, Bentovim A, Goodall G, Hyde C, Lwin R, Sharland E and Elton A (1996) *Child Sexual Abuse: a descriptive and treatment study*. HMSO, London

Aims

To describe those sexually abused children referred to The Hospital for Sick Children, Great Ormond Street, London, and to test whether adding group therapy to family network treatment would lead to better outcome for abused children and their families than family network treatment alone.

Methods

Those referred to Great Ormond Street Hospital over a 19-month period with intra-familial abuse, who were accepted for treatment, were entered into the study; a total of 99 children aged 4–16 years old. From this group 47 children finally entered a randomised controlled trial.

All those entering the randomised controlled trial received the standard family network treatment offered by the hospital team. In addition, half received group therapy.

Selected key results

On objective measures there were no differences between the two treatment groups.

Clinicians rated those who received additional group treatment as having their needs better understood by their carers, and seeing more positive features of themselves.

Strengths of study

Randomised controlled design.

Used some well-validated objective measures.

Limitations of study

Limited to cases of intra-familial abuse referred to a specialist treatment centre, which are unlikely to be representative of sexually abused children as a whole.

Small numbers entered and completed the trial.

The clinician assessments were not conducted 'blind' to treatment group, and were not based on validated measures.

Monck E and New M (1996) *Sexually Abused Children and Adolescents and Young Perpetrators of Sexual Abuse who were Treated in Voluntary Community Facilities.* HMSO, London

Aim

To track the progress made by sexually abused children and adolescents, and young perpetrators through the treatment programmes they had attended in their locality.

Methods

Treatment centres were selected by each of the voluntary agencies taking part in the study, and all young people in the two groups (the sexually abused and the young perpetrators) who attended the centres in 1992 or 1993 were included. They were assessed at the beginning and end of therapy, and 12 months later.

Selected key results

High levels of depression were found for children (66% of over-8 year olds scored high for depression), and their mothers (about half scored over the cut-off point for depression), using checklist measures.

Approximately 10–20% of victims were showing sexualised

behaviour (e.g. making advances to other children or using age-inappropriate sexual language).

Half of the young perpetrators had previously been sexually victimised themselves.

Strengths of study

Outcomes were measured by questionnaires of the children and young people, their parents, teachers and therapists; so a range of perspectives was considered. Some well-validated measures (e.g. CDI, CBCL, *see* page 69) were used to assess mental health and behaviour.

A 'naturalistic' study – trying to study therapy where, and as, it actually happened in real life, rather than in a special clinical research environment.

Limitations of study

At 12-month follow-up there was a very low rate of return of the study questionnaires, and of the therapist assessments. This means that the results may not be representative of the group studied as a whole.

Only children who attended a treatment centre could be included. Only a small proportion of sexually abused children or young perpetrators receive treatment and they may not be representative of the group as a whole. It is not clear how the voluntary agencies selected young people for attendance at the treatment centres.

Sharland E, Seal H, Croucher H, Aldgate J and Jones D (1996) *Professional Intervention in Child Sexual Abuse.* HMSO, London

Aims

To outline the nature of early professional intervention, and to understand the perceptions of children, parents and professionals.

To explore relationships between early interventions and outcomes.

Methods

Stage 1 For all referrals in one county for sexual abuse concerns over a 9-month period, the professional involved was interviewed (220 children referred).

Stage 2 Forty-one children from 34 families were selected for in-depth interview. Thirty-four took part, and the child, parent and professional were all interviewed using a semi-structured interview, including standardised questionnaires.

Stage 3 Thirty-two of these 34 were re-interviewed 12 months later.

Selected key results

High levels of depression, disturbed behaviour and post-traumatic stress disorder were seen in these children. There was no consistent evidence of improvement over time. Depression was strongly linked with remaining at risk of reabuse.

Badly handled initial contact could alienate both the child and parent.

Parents identified that two-thirds of children had unmet needs 12 months after the abuse.

Children abused by outsiders were often given less professional attention after the investigation, and were more likely to have unmet needs.

Strengths of study

A mix of qualitative and quantitative approaches were used. A large amount of useful information was gathered on a sample of children and families, where there was concern about sexual abuse.

Re-interviewing 12 months later meant that children and families were followed through the child protection process.

Limitations of study

Only included children aged 5 and over.

A large proportion of subjects recruited for Stage 2 refused to take part.

Skuse D, Bentovim A, Hodges J, Stevenson J, Andreou C, Lanyado M, New M, Williams B and McMillan D (1998) *The Influence of Early Experience of Sexual Abuse on the Formation of Sexual Preferences during Adolescence.* (Unpublished report and British Medical Journal article[16])

Aims

To assess whether specific personal and experiential influences may increase or decrease the risk of a boy engaging in sexually abusive behaviour, and to examine whether the process that leads boys to become sexual abusers differs according to whether or not they themselves have been victims of sexual abuse.

Methods

Boys were referred by child protection co-ordinators, social work departments and juvenile justice teams. 157 boys were initially surveyed, and 81 of them were assessed in more depth, as were their mothers; 46 of these boys then had detailed psychometric and psychotherapy assessments.

The boys fell into four groups in relation to sexual abuse, allowing two comparisons.

- Victim perpetrators (had been abused themselves and also abused another) were compared to victim non-perpetrators (victim of abuse only), to identify risk factors for sexually abusive behaviour in previously sexually victimised boys.
- Non-victim perpetrators (had abused another, but had not been abused themselves) were compared to antisocial group

(non-victim, non-perpetrators), to identify risk factors for sexually abusive behaviour in non-victimised boys.

Selected key results

Perpetrators of sexual abuse who had themselves been sexually victimised (victim perpetrators) were more likely to report witnessing intra-familial violence than those boys who had been sexually victimised but had not gone on to abuse.

The mothers of non-victim perpetrators had higher rates of having been sexually abused themselves during childhood than mothers of non-victim non-perpetrators (antisocial boys) (63% vs. 13%).

Strengths of study

Very thorough and wide-ranging multi-disciplinary assessments were carried out.

The case–control design allowed for comparisons between the different groups of boys.

Limitations of study

Referrals were from a large specialist centre, so may have comprised more complex and severe cases than the norm.

A number of boys were excluded from the study (for a variety of practical reasons).

Trowell J, Kolvin I, Berelowitz M, Weeramanthri I, Sadowski H, Rushton A, Miles G, Glaser D, Elton A, Rustin M and Hunter M (1998) *Psychotherapy Outcome Study for Sexually Abused Girls*. (Unpublished report)

Aims

To offer group or individual psychotherapy to ameliorate the short- and long-term effects of child sexual abuse.

Establish which symptoms and difficulties respond to which form of psychotherapy.

Methods

100 girls, aged 6–14, who had been sexually abused and currently had symptoms of post-traumatic stress disorder were randomly allocated to two groups:

Group 1 received up to 30 sessions of individual psychoanalytic psychotherapy.

Group 2 received up to 20 sessions of group therapy.

In addition, the sexually abused girls were compared with other non-sexually abused girls referred to the clinic (case–control study).

Selected key results

At the end of treatment there were no major differences found between the two treatment groups. (This is a preliminary finding as the analysis is still underway.)

The sexually abused girls had higher rates of many psychiatric conditions, such as depression and anxiety, than the non-abused girls; and there were higher rates of 'unhealthy functioning' found in their families.

Strengths of study

A randomised controlled study, so the best kind of study to address the aims.

Studied two types of treatment which are commonly suggested for sexually abused children.

Detailed assessments of many different types were carried out by the research team.

Limitations of study

The two groups received different amounts of therapist time (20 vs. 30 sessions) which may influence the results.

Final results are not yet available.

Although it was a large study the numbers of subjects involved may have been too small to show up some subtle differences in effectiveness between the two types of therapy.

Glossary of terms

Abuse-specific and trauma-specific therapies

The term refers to explicitly organising the treatment around the traumatic experience. Successful emotional and cognitive processing of the event(s) is the primary goal. Education is provided about the nature of events and the expected consequences, and children are supported in the appropriate expression of legitimate emotions and behaviours. Interventions are specifically designed to change maladaptive thoughts, feelings, and behaviours associated with the traumatic event.[75]

Cognitive-behaviour therapy (CBT)

A broad range of therapies with a common theme of combining approaches addressing thoughts, and their interactions with behaviour and emotions. Precise measurement of events or symptoms to monitor progress is usually an integral part of the therapy. Several treatment regimes have been formulated specifically for sexually abused children and their parents/carers, and these are described briefly on page 57. For more detailed descriptions of the cognitive behaviour therapies for sexually abused children and their families see Deblinger and Heflin.[72]

Group therapy

Describes any form of therapy which involves a group of people, usually with a similar type of problem, working together with one or two therapists. Different types of therapy can be used in a group setting, and groups using different therapeutic styles are described in the research outlined in this book.

Modelling

The modelling or demonstrating of a desired behaviour by the therapist to help a patient develop new or alternative patterns of behaviour. An example might be where the therapist demonstrates a way of coping in a given social situation.

Psychodynamic therapy

This form of therapy has its recent origins in Freud's work. It attempts to 'approach the patient empathetically from the *inside* in order to help him identify and understand what is happening in his inner world, in relation to his background, upbringing, and development.'[92]

Psychoeducational approach

An approach which is primarily educational, focused on what is known of the psychology of the index problem or phenomena. In the case of child sexual abuse it would include giving accurate information about sexual abuse and its effects and consequences. It would also attempt to correct misconceptions about child sexual abuse and its effects which the child may have.

Post-traumatic stress disorder (PTSD)

A disorder which can follow the experiencing or witnessing of a number of events including violence, disasters and child abuse of all forms. Three types of symptoms occur. First, the traumatic event is re-experienced in the form of intrusive images or dreams. Second, places and objects associated with the event are avoided, and third symptoms of over-arousal such as sleep disturbance and poor concentration are experienced. PTSD is commonly experienced by children who have been sexually abused.

Reactive attachment disorder

This describes specific problems with emotional withdrawal and the forming of safe, close relationships. It can be the result of experiencing abuse.

Social phobia

A fear of being scrutinised in social situations. This leads to high levels of anxiety which can lead to the sufferer avoiding situations where they may meet other people.

Index